Making Sense Sleep Medici

This is a practical and patient-complaint-focused handbook, directed to motivate nonsleep experts and beginners in sleep medicine and technology. This book provides a basic review of the area of sleep, identifies some common patient presentations, and illustrates the types of investigations that should be requested. With sleep and breathing problems being so common and affecting many other chronic clinical conditions, it is important that primary care and other general physicians, as well as allied health practitioners, have a greater appreciation of this area. This text is a valuable go-to handbook for the occasional "sleep" practitioner to refer to.

Key Features:

- Contains specially packaged case scenarios, basic sleep monitoring techniques in detail with sample reports, followed by self-assessment questions.
- Provides direction to health care professionals who encounter patients with sleep and breathing disorders in their practices.
- Uses algorithms and concept maps for dealing with specific symptoms.

Making Sense of

About the Series

The *Making Sense of* series covers a variety of medical topics and subjects allied to medicine. Some of them are practical and technique-based, some provide professional advice, and some relate to professional development. All titles are easy to navigate for quick reference and include plenty of features such as 'summary boxes', 'pearls of wisdom', and 'clinical considerations'. Easy to understand, written in a jargon-free style, and convenient for carrying around, the *Making Sense of* series provides hands-on guidance to be referred to often in both clinical and reference contexts.

Making Sense of Sleep Medicine

A Hands-On Guide

Edited by

Karuna Datta, MD, PhD

FAIMER (GSMC-India), International Sleep Medicine Certification (World Sleep Federation)
Professor, Department of Sports Medicine
Armed Forces Medical College
Pune, Maharashtra, India

Deepak Shrivastava, MD, FAASM, FCCP, FACP, RPSGT

Professor of Medicine, Sleep, Pulmonary and Critical Care
UC Davis School of Medicine
Sacramento, California, USA

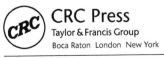

CRC Press
Taylor & Francis Group
Boca Raton London New York

CRC Press is an imprint of the
Taylor & Francis Group, an **informa** business

First edition published 2023
by CRC Press
6000 Broken Sound Parkway NW, Suite 300, Boca Raton, FL 33487–2742

and by CRC Press
4 Park Square, Milton Park, Abingdon, Oxon, OX14 4RN

CRC Press is an imprint of Taylor & Francis Group, LLC

© 2023 Taylor & Francis Group, LLC

ISBN: 978-0-367-55409-5 (hbk)
ISBN: 978-0-367-55408-8 (pbk)
ISBN: 978-1-003-09338-1 (ebk)

DOI: 10.1201/9781003093381

Typeset in Minion
by Apex CoVantage, LLC

This book is dedicated to the memory of my parents, unstinted support of my dear husband, Rakesh, constant encouragement of my lovely sons, Rohan and Ritvik, and priceless companionship of Ginger.

—K.D.

To my better half Kavita and beautiful daughters, Dr. Roopa and her husband Aman Sirohi; and Dr. Richa Shrivastava, for being inspirational to me. My lovely grandchildren Aaryan and Ryanna Sirohi, who always waited to spend just a little time with me.

—D.S.

Contents

Preface

It was April 2019, India, long before the pandemic, when we were planning a session that we were to co-host in a sleep meeting. During the discussions, we pondered on the sleep education programs in progress all over the globe. A glaring gap became evident, and we decided to do something about it. This gap was the relative inadequacy of dealing with sleep complaints and its disorders at the first rung of our health care delivery systems. Yes, at the primary care level! This simple observation mustered our resolve to bridge this gap in our health care systems. The most crucial point we arrived at was the lack of resources specifically targeting sleep and its disorders for health care's clientele.

We set out on a journey to develop educational content including clear explanations of basic concepts, of the commonly seen disorders whereby the patient complains of sleep problems, and of bringing together a suitable management plan. We were very clear that we did not want to complicate the content, but at the same time we sought to ensure that our book would highlight the standards of care and empower practitioners to develop a logical line of reasoning to understand the why and how of comprehensive sleep medicine. Our vision was to bring the concept of sleep medicine under a common umbrella and organize it from the practitioner's point of view, ensuring better communication, management, and clinical outcomes while attending to patients who are often themselves unaware of the detrimental consequences.

And so our journey began . . .

We are glad that, despite the testing times, we could give this book the shape we had envisioned. We hope that our health care fraternity benefits from this book and takes on the formidable task of enabling people to sleep better in this challenging time.

Karuna Datta
Deepak Shrivastava

About the Editors

Col. (Dr.) Karuna Datta, MD, PhD

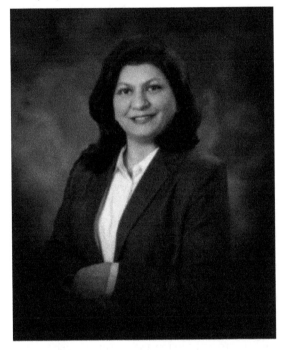

Karuna Datta is a 1994 medical graduate from the Armed Forces Medical College, Pune, India. She completed her MD (Physiology) in December 2002 and DNB (Physiology) from the National Board of Education, Delhi, in 2003. Her journey in sleep medicine started as a WHO Fellow in 2007 when she worked in the Neurophysiology Lab at NIMHANS Bangalore. Further, she did two weeks of observership in sleep medicine at the Division of Sleep Medicine, Harvard Medical School, and Brighams and Women Hospital, Boston, USA, in 2008. She completed two years (2009–2011) of medical education fellowship from the Foundation of Advancement in Medical Education and Research (FAIMER) regional center at Mumbai, India. She has cleared the International Sleep Medicine Certification Examination from the World Sleep Society in 2012. Karuna Datta was awarded her PhD in 2016 for her work on "Electrophysiological Characterisation of Yoga Nidra and Its Role in Insomnia' from AIIMS, New Delhi, India.

Her association with the National Sleep Medicine Course at India spans more than a decade when she not only contributed actively to designing the course curriculum but was also a key person in its roll out.

She has a keen interest in medical education and a passion for promotion of sleep in the community and among sleep professionals. She has authored a book, *My Sleep Diary: Reflections Within and Beyond*, which has been written for a layperson not only to know about one's sleep but also to identify when to seek medical help.

She presently is a principal investigator of the Government of India–funded project in Yoga Nidra and Cognition and continues her passion for yoga nidra.

This book is an attempt to reach out to all health professionals with an aim to simplify the diagnosis and management of sleep disorders at the primary care level. It is her belief that sleep practice using recommended guidelines at that level can not only improve patient's sleep but also reduce the disease burden of the associated disorders.

Deepak Shrivastava, MD, FAASM, FCCP, FACP, CMD, HMDC

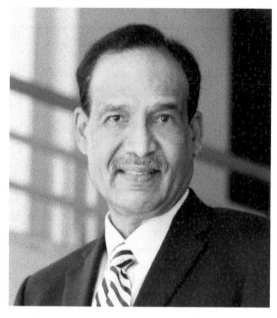

Deepak Shrivastava has practiced medicine in the United States for the last 40 years. He received his clinical education at Brooklyn Jewish Hospital, New York, and University of California at Davis. He is a Fellow of AASM, AACP, and ACP.

He is Professor of Internal Medicine, Sleep Medicine, Pulmonary, and Critical Care at UC Davis School of Medicine and faculty at UC Davis affiliated SJGH. He is senior faculty at the Sleep Medicine Fellowship Program at UC Davis. He is Adjunct Professor of Pharmacy at University of Pacific, School of Pharmacy and Assistant Professor of Medicine at St. George's School of Medicine. He is Assistant Professor of Medicine at School of Osteopathic Medicine in Vallejo, California, and Associate Medical Director for a California managed care organization.

He received his sleep medicine training at Stanford. He is board certified in all his specialties, as well as long-term and post–acute medicine and hospice medicine. He is the recipient of many academic and service awards. He has received the 2015 Medical Director of the year award of the American Medical Directors Association and the Lifetime Achievement Award for educational endeavors internationally. His biography was released in 2017, commemorating his work around the world for the education of professionals and public.

He is an active researcher with a keen interest in medical education. He is directly involved in health care quality and performance improvement throughout his career. In addition to his active practice of pulmonary, critical care, and sleep medicine in an ACGME-accredited residency program, since 1989 he is involved in hospice care and long-term care. He is a member of the National Partnership for Healthcare and Hospice Innovation (NPHI). He actively works to influence health care policy at both the political and the administrative levels.

For over three decades, he has been involved in the education of medical students, house staff, fellows, physicians, dentists, nurses, respiratory therapists, and, more importantly, with many community organizations. He has directed multiple Mechanical Ventilation, Pulmonary Function, and Sleep Medicine Courses since 1999.

He is an inventor and author and has a keen interest in medical education. He works with local, national, and international organizations and has a long record of public service. He creates and publishes both scientific and public education content regularly.

He believes in translating and applying scientific principles to daily life. His quote "any science that does not relate to daily life is not mature enough and is only work in progress" truly reflects his belief and values. He is a believer in "360 degrees of life," a philosophy that must be embedded in the practice of medicine to make living a wholesome experience!

Dr. Shrivastava believes that life is not only about high-quality cognitive wakefulness for 16 hours and restful and restorative sleep for 8. It is about living each moment with nonexhaustive capacity to capture the joy of living a beautiful human life every day. It takes in psychological, behavioral, spiritual, cultural, religious, and social dimensions: the organism as a whole!

Deepak Shrivastava enjoys reading, writing, playing music, tennis, skiing, backpacking, and occasionally just not doing anything.

Contributors

EDITORS

Deepak Shrivastava, MD, FAASM, FCCP, FACP, RPSGT
Professor of Medicine, Sleep, Pulmonary, and
Critical Care
UC Davis School of Medicine
Sacramento, California, USA

Karuna Datta, MD, PhD
FAIMER (GSMC-India), International Sleep
Medicine Certification (World Sleep
Federation-2012)
Professor
Department of Sports Medicine
Armed Forces Medical College
Pune, Maharashtra, India

CONTRIBUTORS

Ajitpal Sethi, MD, FAASM, ABMS
Assistant Professor of Medicine and Sleep Medicine
UC Davis School of Medicine
Sacramento, California, USA
Sleep Specialist, Sutter Gould Medical Foundation
Stockton, California, USA

Deepak Shrivastava, MD, FAASM, FCCP, FACP, RPSGT
Professor of Medicine, Sleep, Pulmonary, and
Critical Care
UC Davis School of Medicine
Sacramento, California, USA

Karuna Datta, MD, PhD
FAIMER (GSMC-India), International Sleep
Medicine Certification (World Sleep
Federation-2012)
Professor
Department of Sports Medicine
Armed Forces Medical College
Pune, Maharashtra, India

Richa Shrivastava, MD
Department of Internal Medicine
San Joaquin General Hospital
Stockton, California, USA

Thomas Joseph, MD
Department of Sports Medicine
Armed Forces Medical College
Pune, Maharashtra, India

PART 1

Basics First

Basic Physiology of Sleep

KARUNA DATTA

INTRODUCTION

Understanding the physiology of sleep helps a physician in several ways. First, it helps the physician to enable the patient to understand about how a particular disease occurs. This doctor–patient communication is more effective and convincing when the doctor himself understands the pathology in respect to the physiology of a particular disorder. Second, it can help the physician tailor the approach to the disorder and modify treatment strategies according to the patient's requirement. Normal human sleep is an active process. It has two distinct types—NREM and REM—with clearly differentiating features and physiology. This understanding of physiology also helps in the research and development in the area of sleep assessment and in the development of innovative therapies for sleep problems and disorders.

WHY SHOULD A PRIMARY CARE PHYSICIAN KNOW ABOUT THE PHYSIOLOGY OF SLEEP?

- Understanding the differences between the physiology of wakefulness, NREM sleep, and REM sleep is required at times to correlate the patient symptoms that may occur during one or all phases. For example, the relatively increased incidence of cardiac events in REM can be explained by the physiology of REM sleep and autonomic interaction with the cardiovascular system.

- The physician can also correlate clinically the effects of sleep deprivation better once the physiology of sleep and circadian rhythm and physiology in sleep is comprehended. The physiology of circadian rhythm and physiology in sleep are covered in subsequent chapters.

- The assessment of sleep is done using multiple sensors, and various physiological parameters are recorded. The polysomnography report can be better analyzed once the physician understands the various physiological changes expected during sleep. A keen eye can pick up some early signs of a disease. For example, an occurrence of a short-duration arrythmia during the night at a time when patient complains of night sweats and palpitations may warrant a cardiovascular workup for an early diagnosis. Similarly, increased frequency of unexplained microarousals at night might alert the physician to look for evidence of coexisting desaturations, arrythmias, respiratory disturbances, or something entirely of a spontaneous nature to further categorize the disorder.

DOI: 10.1201/9781003093381-2

HISTORICAL PERSPECTIVE

Hans Berger, in his experiments in the 1920s, had explained that surface potentials from the scalp indicate the status of the brain. He also propounded that these potentials change in their amplitude and frequency over time, determining the brain state. Later experiments by Bremer in the 1930s and by Moruzzi and Magoun in 1940s deduced that the anterior areas of the brain stem, when stimulated, caused arousal and that its lesion affected the sleep-wake state of the experimental animal. Lesions of the basal forebrain precluded slow wave sleep, and these areas were inhibited by noradrenergic stimulation. Electrical stimulation of the basal forebrain caused slow wave sleep. Experiments by Michel Jouvet helped identify small neuronal groups in the pons and medulla that caused brain activation, muscle atonia, and REM sleep. In 1953, Aserinsky and Kleitman proved the duality of sleep, which is two types: rapid eye movement (REM) and non-REM (NREM). Early contributions of Christian Guilleminault and Haurii & Orr gave shape to present-day sleep medicine.

NORMAL HUMAN SLEEP

Sleep primarily depends on two processes. First, one considers the time since the last sleep period, or Process S, which is also related to the increase in sleep deficit or sleep debt, which builds with deprivation and dissipates with sleep. It is proportional to the duration of prior wakefulness. The second process depends on the circadian rhythm of sleep and wake propensity, i.e., Process C. The difference between the two drives sleep, or the homeostatic drive of sleep. Most conditions can be explained by these two processes except a few that still cannot be explained. One among them is the sleep inertia that one sees immediately after waking up from a full night's sleep.

Normal human sleep on average is approximately 7–9 hours, which decreases with aging. The requirement is much greater as a neonate or infant, being approximately 16–18 hours and then decreases to 8–10 hours by the time of teens or adolescence. By the age of 4–5 years, the child starts having most of sleep at nighttime and in a single uninterrupted episode. At nighttime, sleep is continuous in adults, and 75–90% of the total sleep time is NREM sleep and 10–20% is REM sleep. The

NREM and REM types of sleep alternate in cycles, each cycle lasting around 90–110 minutes. In the earlier cycles, NREM sleep predominates. REM sleep duration increases as the sleep cycle progresses toward the wake-up time. **When a person's sleep duration is reduced, REM sleep is deprived more.**

NREM sleep has various stages: I, II, III, and IV. Stage II NREM sleep is characterized by sleep spindles and K-complexes. Stages III and IV comprise slow wave sleep. During this sleep, delta waves in EEG are seen, and they have a frequency of 0.5–4 Hz. REM sleep is also called paradoxical sleep due to the similarity of EEG to the wake state type, which is of low amplitude and high frequency. REM sleep has characteristic bursts of rapid eye movements. There is intense muscle hypotonia in the rest of the body except for the muscles of the diaphragm required for respiration and the eye movement muscles. This intense muscle hypotonia in the body, as seen in EMG, with rapid eye movements is characteristic of REM sleep.

UNDERSTANDING SLEEP AND ITS DISORDERS

Sleep was initially considered a passive phenomenon. It was believed that the state of sleep occurred when the inputs to keep awake were reduced. Experiments showed that deafferentation or a lesion in the ascending reticular activating system caused insomnia; hence the sensory inputs were thought to be responsible for being awake and, when they were reduced, a sleep state ensued. It was by von Economo, an Austrian psychiatrist who observed patients of Encephalitis lethargica during the swine flu epidemic in the early twentieth century. He found two types of clinical presentations of these patients: one who showed insomnia-like features and another who had ophthalmoplegia and extreme somnolence. His detailed notes brought out this stark difference in the two clinical presentation types very lucidly. On necropsy of these patients, it was found that the two types of sleep symptoms, i.e., insomnia and somnolence, had distinctly different anatomical lesions, i.e., lesions in the posterior and anterior hypothalamus, respectively. The ones with drowsiness also had oculomotor nerve nuclei lesion, explaining the ophthalmoplegia associated with these cases. This was a definite indication of distinct sleep-wake regions in the brain, the lesion of which produced insomnia and extreme somnolence, respectively.

The reduction in activation of the brain stem reticular core formation induces sleep. Electrical stimulation of this area can cause arousal and awaken a sleeping animal. Various pathways run parallel to this core region. Cholinergic, serotonergic, noradrenergic, and dopaminergic pathways are known to affect the sleep-wake state. Diffuse cholinergic connections in the pathways connected to the basal forebrain are seen to be stimulated at the time of arousal. Acetylcholine antagonists are found to have effects on sleep by inducing and prolonging sleep. Similarly, muscarinic acetylcholine antagonists also have sedative effects. Tricyclic antidepressants, which are anticholinergic, are used for treating insomnia.

Benzodiazepine binds to GABA-A receptors and facilitates sleep. Benzodiazepines facilitate sleep but reduce deep sleep, and hence the patient often complains of reduced quality despite increased duration. Zolpidem binds to a subset of benzodiazepine receptors and promotes sleep without affecting deep sleep, thereby improving the quality of sleep in patients.

A lesion in raphe nuclei (the serotonergic pathway) produces sleep and 5HT agonists promote sleep. Serotonin reuptake inhibitors reduce REM sleep, and dopamine reuptake blockers produce arousal. The activity of noradrenergic neurons in the locus coeruleus is related to the tasks of attention. Loss of muscle atonia is found with very small lesions ventral to the locus coeruleus. Antihistamines cause inhibition of thalamic neurons causing sedative effects. These experiments give a clue that distinct regions of brain are involved in the NREM, REM, and wake states.

Drugs like benzodiazepines and zolpidem, which modulate their action through GABA-ergic action, are used for promoting sleep. Excessive daytime sleepiness of narcolepsy is treated with amphetamines as it causes the release and inhibit the uptake of catecholamines. The cataplexy of narcolepsy is managed with tricyclic antidepressants due to its inhibition of uptake of noradrenaline and serotonin, hence inhibiting REM muscle atonia.

Modafinil is a weak dopamine reuptake inhibitor and releases orexin and histamine from the lateral hypothalamus and tuberomammillary nucleus, respectively, causing increased arousal.

Drugs that affect arousal can also act via modulating Process C by altering the melatonin levels like ramelteon, which is a melatonin agonist.

Distinct centers for sleep and wakefulness exist, and sleep is an active phenomenon. Various cortical and subcortical areas are involved in the generation and maintenance of sleep and wake states. Work by Saper's group postulated a proposal for the relatively clear demarcation of NREM, REM, and wake states. They proposed that a flip-flop model makes the transitions smooth and that the intrusion of one state is not allowed into another due to this mechanism. The proposal mentions a sleep-wake switch, a REM-NREM switch, and the stability of the transitions enforced by orexin neurons. The sleep-wake switch describes the wake-promoting neurons from the brain stem. Cholinergic, monoaminergic, and glutamatergic neurons provide direct and indirect innervation via the thalamus to the hypothalamus, cerebral cortex, and basal part of the forebrain. The orexin neurons in the lateral hypothalamus reinforce these and directly stimulate the cerebral cortex and basal forebrain to maintain arousal. The primary sleep-promoting area in the ventrolateral preoptic (VLPO) and median preoptic areas in the hypothalamus inhibits these arousal pathways. The arousal system can also directly inhibit the VLPO causing a sudden and rapid transition from sleep to wake. This acts as a flip-flop switch, where the VLPO can inhibit arousal pathways, which can inhibit VLPO.

The transition between REM and NREM is also explained by such a flip-flop switch between REM-on and REM-off neurons and NREM-generating neurons. These are also under the control of monoaminergic and cholinergic pathways, again causing rapid transitions between NREM and REM sleep. The monoaminergic neurons inhibit VLPO during wake and inhibit REM-on neurons and excite REM-off neurons to prevent the intrusion of REM into wake. Orexin neurons play an important role here in the stabilization of this switch. Orexin neurons are found to be affected with low levels of hypocretin in cases of narcolepsy. Patients with narcolepsy have sudden REM episodes during wake, sleep fragmentation at night, excessive daytime sleepiness, sleep paralysis, and cataplexy due to the lack of the stabilizing effect of the descending motor inhibitory control, causing muscle atonia during the wake state in narcolepsy. These patients also have hypnagogic or hypnopompic hallucination that occur at sleep onset and at sleep offset.

NREM and REM have differences not only in the EEG characteristics as previously described, but the body physiology also is different. NREM constitutes approximately 75% of the sleep cycles in adults and 50% in infants. The stage shows reduced heart rate, slower respiration, reduction in blood pressure, reduced muscle tone, and sympathetic nerve activity as compared to the wake state. The cerebral blood flow remains similar, and a slight increase in airway resistance is seen as compared to the wake state. Temperature regulation is maintained but at lower set points as compared to wake. As compared to NREM, REM sleep is characterized by increased and irregular heart rate, irregular respiration, fluctuating blood pressure, and sympathetic nerve activity is also found to have fluctuations with episodic increases. The airway resistance further increases and becomes irregular as compared to NREM sleep. Cerebral blood flow, compared to NREM sleep, is increased, and energy expenditure is higher. The body temperature is not regulated, and it starts to drift toward the local environment. Penile erections in males is documented during REM sleep. Assessment of male penile erections during REM sleep can be used to differentiate between psychological and physiological impotence.

Dreams are documented in both NREM sleep and REM sleep but are very different in nature. Dreams during REM sleep are reported to be vivid, more visual, longer, and with more emotional content. In contrast, NREM dreams are more conceptual, shorter, and less visual, with reduced or negligible emotional content.

FUNCTIONS OF SLEEP

A lot about the functions of sleep are known from sleep deprivation studies. Sleep deprivation in an individual is associated with reduced performance, irritability, lack of concentration, and sleepiness. This deprivation also makes the subject prone to infections, impairs memory, and hastens the onset of various disorders. Energy conservation, improvement in physical and mental health, enhancement of immunity, improved memory, better decision making, and increased concentration are known to occur when deprivation is reverted. Studies show that sleep causes learning and improvement in cognitive function. Sleep is also known to have a bidirectional relationship with emotions, implying correlations of better mood with good sleep and of irritability and feeling "low" with sleep deprivation. Sleep deprivation affects the release and function of gonadal hormones. Effects on the hypothalamic hypopituitary axis impairs body metabolism, growth, gonadal function, feeding habits, and mood. More information on endocrinal changes during sleep is given in Chapter 3, where the physiological changes during sleep are discussed in detail.

Studies show that stress manifests with an individual's susceptibility. Some have increased blood pressure, and some may show sleep initiation and maintenance insomnia. Similarly some individuals suffer more circadian disruption compared to others, though with the same amount of intermeridian travel. Individual susceptibility to sleep loss is also documented, and hence a physician might find some people in a group of similar sleep profiles doing worse or having more symptoms than others after being deprived of sleep. Awareness about individual susceptibility to sleep loss is important for a physician since early detection and treatment help the patient, and one can suitably educate and motivate the individual earlier to prevent future occurrences.

CONCLUSION

Alterations in physiology can be picked up early when one is aware of the pathophysiological process of the disorder and can help in early diagnosis and management.

With long-standing sleep deprivation or impaired sleep, the individual might be at an increased risk for cardiovascular and metabolic disorders, which can be monitored or diagnosed earlier if the physician is aware of the possibilities.

Awareness of physiology also helps us in the management of disorders by explaining to the patient and motivating the patient to control the disease. For example, in cases of circadian rhythm disorders, there is a need of an awareness talk with patients on the importance of maintaining biorhythms, light exposure, and the care to be taken before sleep time while managing their sleep. Another example is the practice of explaining to the chronic insomnia patient the fact that there are distinct sleep and wake centers. Many patients with chronic insomnia are on long-standing drugs, and they often insist on drug prescriptions. Apart from educating them about the side effects of long-term drug intake, it is required to motivate them toward an additional nonpharmacological approach. It helps them to explain about how these drugs act by activating the sleep centers. This can only act as a support for a chronic insomnia patient. It cannot by itself treat the condition because the actual pathophysiology is more of heightened arousal; i.e., something is required to quieten the wake centers, and nothing is wrong in the generation of sleep. This self-motivates the patient to start taking sleep hygiene, stimulus control, relaxation exercises, and cognitive behavioral therapy more seriously. The function of good-quality sleep in better learning, memory, and critical decision making, compared to a deprived state, is especially important for students and high performers. Awareness of the physiology of sleep and physiology in sleep improves doctor–patient communication as a whole and makes it more meaningful and insightful.

SUGGESTED READING

1. Barrett KE, Boitano S, Barman SM, Brooks HL, Ganong WF, editors. *Ganong's Review of Medical Physiology*. 25th ed. New York, NY: McGraw-Hill; 2015. 768 p. (A Lange medical book).

2

Physiology of Circadian Rhythm

KARUNA DATTA

INTRODUCTION

The master clock of the circadian rhythm resides in the hypothalamus, and the suprachiasmatic nucleus is the master controller. This nucleus has molecular clock mechanisms that can be entrained by various photic and nonphotic stimuli. Peripheral clocks in the body in non-SCN tissues are in alignment with the master clock; however, some stimuli can uncouple the master clock from the peripheral clocks in the non-SCN tissues. In this chapter, the basic concept of the master clock mechanism, as well as its coupling or uncoupling with the peripheral clocks, is explained, and the physiology of the circadian rhythm has been laid out with specific emphasis on the various physiological mechanisms that can help in the assessment and management of circadian rhythm disorders.

WHY IS THE CIRCADIAN RHYTHM PHYSIOLOGY IMPORTANT FOR UNDERSTANDING SLEEP AND CIRCADIAN RHYTHM DISORDERS?

- Process C and Process S make up a two-process sleep-wake model proposed by Alexander Borberly. Process S is a sleep-wake-dependent homeostatic process and circadian process; Process C interacts with Process S. Their interaction results in the sleep and wake timing and determines the sleep drive.

- Circadian rhythm has a distinct pathway and is primarily entrained by light. The role of nonphotic stimuli on the circadian rhythm is also emerging, and hence both photic and nonphotic stimuli affect the circadian rhythm in the body.

DOI: 10.1201/9781003093381-3

- Not only does it have an important role in sleep-wake regulation, but the master clock, suprachiasmatic nucleus interacts with peripheral clocks in the organs and tissues to promote homeostasis.

- The role of its interaction on the endocrinal system, behavioral changes, cognition, and body metabolism is vital to understand pathophysiology and treatment for many disorders. A new concept of so-called circadian medicine has emerged in the recent past that highlights the role of the circadian system in pathophysiology and the management of disorders. The importance of the circadian light-dark cycle in ICU settings has been emphasized for healthier outcomes of patients admitted in ICU and wards.

- In today's clinical practice, circadian rhythm sleep disorders are commonly encountered. The physiology of circadian rhythm is complex but is important to understand its disorders and the interaction with other systems in health and disease.

WHAT IS THE CIRCADIAN RHYTHM MECHANISM? UNDERSTANDING THE MOLECULAR CLOCK MECHANISM

Circadian rhythm means "around a day," and the inherent rhythm approximates slightly more than 24 hours. The rhythm is generated due to a molecular clock mechanism. The master clock is situated in the suprachiasmatic nucleus present in the hypothalamus. The master clock interacts with peripheral clocks that are present in the various organs and tissues.

The basis of the molecular clock mechanism comes from transcription translation feedback loops (TTFL). These TTFL are found in the suprachiasmatic (SCN) nucleus and non-SCN tissue.

Brain and muscle Arnt-like 1 (BMAL-1), circadian locomotor output cycles kaput (CLOCK), cryptochrome (Cry), and period (Per) genes are the most important for the molecular clock mechanism.

The TTFL mechanism is explained in Figure 2.1. The diagram representing TTFL has been made very simplistic to make it easy to understand. The various points as marked f1–5 in the diagram are further elaborated here:

1. Transcription factors BMAL-1 and CLOCK dimerize in the cytoplasm.
2. These dimers then enter the nucleus, bind to Cry and Per genes, and promote transcription, causing an expression of PER and CRY proteins.
3. These proteins also dimerize and inhibit the transcriptional effects of BMAL-1 and CLOCK proteins. Both PER and CRY proteins peak

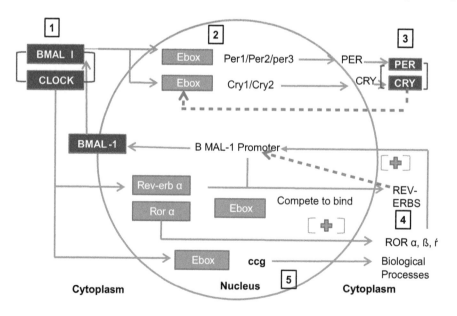

Figure 2.1 Basics of transcription translation feedback loop.

at dusk and activate clock-controlled genes and inhibit BMAL-1 and CLOCK proteins. Casein kinase 1 epsilon (CK1ε) inhibits post-translational nuclear translocation of PER and CRY proteins, and they also tag them for degradation by phosphorylating these proteins. Therefore, CK1 regulates PER stability.

4. RAR- related orphan receptors (ROR) play an important role in circadian rhythm. RORα positively regulates expression of BMAL-1 thus maintaining the circadian rhythm. BMAL-1 is made available by the positive feedback (TTFL) loops. Along with RORs, which activate transcription, another set of nuclear receptors called REV-ERBS inhibit transcription. The REV-ERBα expression is regulated by BMAL-1. RORs and REV-ERBs are expressed in an oscillatory manner, leading to the alternating activation and repression of BMAL-1 expression.

5. Also seen in the diagram is the effect of CLOCK protein on clock-controlled genes (CCG) in the transcription of various proteins.

SCN receives afferents from the limbic system and from areas of the thalamus and hypothalamus, apart from the retina, and hence has both photic and nonphotic inputs. Some of the areas like the dorsomedial nucleus of hypothalamus (DMH) and intergeniculate lamina (IGL) of the thalamus also receive nonphotic stimuli directly or indirectly and communicate with SCN where SCN sends its afferents and receives efferent from these areas. Studies show that IGL plays an important role in the regulation of nonphotic regulation of circadian rhythm by stimulating arousal inputs. Serotonergic pathways via the Raphe nuclei are known to modulate SCN effects and to mediate nonphotic effects too. DMH neurons activate areas in lateral hypothalamus promoting arousal. DMH is known to inhibit areas in the ventrolateral preoptic areas that inhibit the ascending arousal system, thus promoting arousal. The circadian rhythm of activity states, meal timings, and cortisol are found to be eliminated following lesions of the DMH.

INTERRELATIONSHIP OF SCN MASTER CLOCK WITH THE PERIPHERY

The master clock is primarily entrained by light. Photic inputs fall on the retina, and via the retino-hypothalamic tract, these inputs reach the master clock situated in the suprachiasmatic nucleus. This pathway has melanopsin-containing ganglion cells, distinctly different from the optic pathway. Studies show that disruption of both rods and cones keeps the circadian inputs intact via this pathway. Light causes glutamate secretion in the SCN. Retino-hypothalamic-tract-mediated glutamate signaling in the SCN causes CREB-mediated transcription of Per genes. Per gene expression is inhibited by arousal. The role of PER proteins in molecular clocks has been explained earlier.

Photic input also reaches the IGL, which has an indirect pathway to SCN. The role of light can be further understood by the fact that it is associated with melatonin suppression. Photic suppression of melatonin can be caused by 460 nm light. The blue light range of the light spectrum is extremely sensitive. This is the spectrum also commonly seen at nighttime in modern households. Delayed work timings or delayed sleep times with exposure to light at night is enough to cause changes in the rhythm. Under normal circumstances, there is a dim light melatonin onset (DLMO). Melatonin hormone secretion fluctuates with seasonal variations depending on the duration of day-night pattern. It is released from the pineal gland and acts on its receptors to promote sleepiness and reduction in sleep onset latency. It reinforces the synchronization of the circadian clock and acts as a time giver. Exogenous melatonin, if given before the endogenous secretion, causes an advance phase, promoting sleepiness. Melatonin administration in the evening thus induces sleepiness in insomniacs and can be prescribed in patients with jet lag syndrome to help normalize their deranged circadian rhythm. Melatonin receptor agonists have also been tried for similar effects. The American Association of Sleep Medicine guidelines for melatonin use in inducing sleep are described in individual chapters regarding the management of various sleep disorders later in the book.

The master clock is required for the peripheral clock to be kept in phase synchrony. Synchronization of the central and peripheral clocks is also responsible for the modulating function of other systems like the neurohormonal system, cardiovascular system, reproduction, immunity, etc. On the other hand, it can also be modified by inputs of blood glucose, feeding, temperature, etc. Certain inputs of feeding, social cues, activity states can uncouple the peripheral clock from the master clock

The circadian cues and its integration with physiological processes prepare the system in anticipation, e.g., for a human, of the availability of food more during daytime, and there is an understanding that neuroendocrinal responses enhance this environmental influence. Endogenous rhythms in adipose tissue and the liver can be synchronized by SCN, keeping it aligned to the day and night cycle. Studies show that lipoprotein kinase regulation by the adipose tissue and blood glucose regulation in the liver may be altered. In cases where untimely feeding at night happens, the peripheral clock may uncouple to the SCN coupling of the day-night pattern due to its modulation by the blood levels of blood glucose and other nutrients. Light entrains SCN. Hence prolonged lighting at night, decreased light time in the winter, or a phase shift of light-dark cycles as in transmeridian travel may appear innocuous but might lead to subtle negative effects that are within our control. Avoiding them and being able to correct them may help in promoting better health and lifestyle.

PHYSIOLOGICAL VARIABLES THAT HELP IN ASSESSMENT OF CIRCADIAN RHYTHM

- Experimental studies can be done using constant routine protocols and free running protocols. Depending on the requirements of the study, various other indicators of sleep habit, and feeding time, activity monitors using videography, actigraphy, etc. may be used. Actigraphy and a minimum of 2 weeks of sleep logs/diary are recommended to study circadian rhythm.
- Core body temperature and plasma cortisol and melatonin levels may indicate circadian rhythm.
- Determination of the core body temperature minimum (CBT_{min}) is important for planning therapeutic modalities using light and exercise. Stimulus just after the CBT_{min} causes phase advance, and stimulus just before CBT_{min} causes phase delay. CBT_{min} happens usually 3 hours before the habitual wake period. Its determination is extremely vital in diagnosing and treating circadian rhythm disorders discussed in Chapter 13.

- Melatonin estimation may be used to determine dim light melatonin onset (DLMO). Understanding physiology and actions of melatonin helps in exogenous melatonin administration in disorders. For further details on melatonin and its prescription for disorders, please refer to Chapter 13.

USE OF PROCESS C AND PROCESS S IN PREDICTING ALERTNESS AND PERFORMANCE

Prediction of alertness and performance is done by the use of inputs regarding sleep-wake. The inputs required to predict alertness are the timing of work hours with or without sleep hours, amount of prior sleep, and duration of prior wake (i.e., both circadian and homeostatic), summed. These can then predict:

- Alertness and psychomotor performance.
- Level at which risk of alertness/performance impairment starts.
- Sleep onset latency.
- Time of awakening from sleep.

CIRCADIAN AND PHYSIOLOGICAL FUNCTION: GENES AND DISEASE CORRELATIONS AND BASIS FOR THERAPEUTICS

A disrupted gene of the molecular clock mechanism is associated with varied physiological effects. Abnormal gluconeogenesis is associated with gene disruption of BMAL-1 and CLOCK, abnormal lipogenesis with the BMAL-1 gene and with metabolic syndrome with disruption of the CLOCK gene, altered sleep pattern with BMAL-1, Cry1, Cry2, and Clock genes. Abnormal apoptosis is found with disruption of Per1 and Per2 genes. Progressive arthropathy and infertility are also seen with disruption of the BMAL-1 gene. Similarly, abnormal bone metabolism and cerebellar ataxia are associated with disruption of the Rorα gene, and locomotor difficulties, retinal degeneration, and male reproductive abnormality during the first six months of age are seen with disruption of Rorβ gene. Sleep phase syndromes may be found to be advanced or delayed as seen with disruption of the Per genes.

The circadian rhythm has a potential to induce physiological changes and vice versa. In the coming era, this role may be substantially explored. Emerging results show promising value of the role of light as therapy in psychiatric disorders and in circadian rhythm disorders like delayed sleep-wake phase disorder, jet lag, shift work, etc. The role of circadian rhythm disruption in predisposing for psychiatric disorder is also documented. Physical exercise in the morning has been known to advance sleep, and exercise very near bedtime delays sleep. Circadian prescriptions modulating feeding time, activity schedules, and light exposure have been tried to overcome jet-lag-related dips in alertness and cognitive performance. Similarly, the prevention of disorders or further aggravation of disorders, e.g., metabolic disorders, may be prevented by timely sleep and feeding habits and a healthy exercise schedule at the right time of the day.

A regular sleep time, a healthy feeding time, and avoidance of social activity or media time near bedtime have shown to be promising adjuncts in therapy for the delayed sleep phase syndromes seen in adolescents. Parents, if aware about the need of sleep-wake discipline, may be able to prevent circadian rhythm disorders in their children at a subclinical level itself, thus preventing its emergence as a disorder.

The circadian system and sleep-wake regulation converge to promote a milieu conducive for growth and better well-being. Thyroid-stimulating hormone, which stimulates the secretion of thyroid hormones, is regulated by the circadian rhythm. Sleep opposes this rhythm and inhibits the release of TSH. Sleep is known to increase the release of growth hormone, parathyroid hormone, and prolactin. This effect of circadian rhythm on sleep and the effects of sleep on the circadian rhythm highlight the importance in its synchrony. The desynchronization of the peripheral clocks from the master clock with cues related to metabolism, behavior, attention, and arousal state poses a challenge for homeostasis. These may be indicators of the progression of disease, and physiological interventions using bright light exposure, avoidance of light exposure, feed time alterations, and social activity offer a potent recipe for a nonpharmacological prescription approach for the prevention of disease and treatment as well.

CONCLUSION

The suprachiasmatic nucleus is the master circadian clock and regulates various peripheral clocks in the tissues. Light is the most important factor that can entrain this rhythm via the distinct retino-hypothalamic thalamic pathway. Nonphotic stimuli, like food intake and social rhythm, can uncouple the regulation of the peripheral clock from the master clock. The change in rhythm may predispose the individual to various disorders. Assessing circadian rhythm markers helps in planning circadian prescriptions, and using circadian prescriptions to help restore circadian rhythm can promote patient well-being.

SUGGESTED READING

1. Datta K. Biological rhythm and neuropsychiatric disorders. In Sleep and Neuropsychiatric Disorders [Internet], edited by R Gupta, DN Neubauer, SR Pandi-Perumal. Singapore: Springer Nature Singapore; 2022 [cited 2022 May 18]. pp. 53–63. https://link.springer.com/10.1007/978-981-16-0123-1_3.

3

Physiological Changes during Sleep

KARUNA DATTA

INTRODUCTION

The sleep stages are distinctly different in their EEG characteristics and in the physiological changes that occur during them. This chapter introduces the need-to-know physiology during sleep from a clinician's perspective and highlights important physiological changes seen during sleep. Certain physiological concepts may be repeated later while explaining the pathophysiology of some disorders for better understanding. Various changes in the cardiovascular system and its interaction with the autonomic system, endocrine system, metabolism, and brain are described here. Respiratory physiology is described in detail in Chapter 4. The clinical relevance of understanding physiological changes is brought out and further explained, keeping in mind the various assessment techniques utilized in sleep studies.

THE NEED-TO-KNOW PHYSIOLOGICAL CHANGES DURING SLEEP

As a primary care physician or any health care practitioner, the utility of understanding physiology in sleep is primarily to:

- Help evaluate sleep disorders
- Correlate the symptoms and identify possible etiology
- Better understand the reports of polysomnography, MSLT, actigraphy, sleep diary and other sleep assessment tools
- Communicate the pathophysiology of the disorder such as to motivate the patient to follow principles for good sleep
- Make assessment more robust using a combination of various tools especially in locations

DOI: 10.1201/9781003093381-4

- where there are long waiting lists or access to sleep labs is difficult
- Be able to identify red flag signs to prioritize referrals to various specialists for ongoing treatment

PHYSIOLOGICAL CHANGES DURING SLEEP

Sleep affects physiology of almost all body systems. We discuss them here under the following broad areas:

- Effects of sleep on the cardiovascular system and its interaction with the autonomic system
- Effects of sleep on the respiratory system (this is dealt with separately in Chapter 4)
- Effects of sleep on the endocrine system and metabolism
- Effects of sleep on neurological processing, the brain, and higher cognitive function.
- Other effects of sleep

EFFECTS OF SLEEP ON CARDIOVASCULAR SYSTEM AND ITS INTERACTION WITH AUTONOMIC SYSTEM

The cardiovascular and autonomic systems interact during sleep. Under normal conditions, parasympathetic drive starts to occur before sleep onset, and the reduction in sympathetic drive, as noted by muscle sympathetic nerve activity (MSNA), is seen with a deepening of sleep. This may be an important attribute for normal sleep, since problems initiating sleep are very commonly associated with increased presleep arousal.

During the initial stages of sleep, there is an overall parasympathetic predominance, and baroreceptor gain is high, leading to stability of blood pressure. Usually, a dip in blood pressure of approximately 10% during NREM sleep is found. In fact, cases that show less than 10% dip in night blood pressure are called non-Dippers and have been found to have an increased risk for cardiovascular mortality, arrythmias, myocardial infarction, etc. MSNA is almost half in slow wave sleep as compared to being awake.

At the time of transit between NREM to REM, bursts of vagal nerve activity are seen that might cause a sudden reduction of heart rate, and thus asystole is commonly seen. With the onset of REM, heart rate and blood pressure begin to rise and often fluctuate. Patients with coronary artery disease, postmyocardial infarction, and diabetes are found to have a higher sympathetic drive during sleep compared to normal volunteers. This increase is further stepped up during REM sleep.

The effect of the sympathetic drive on the heart causes an increase in heart rate (chronotropic), increased excitability (bathmotropic), increased contractility (ionotropic), increased conduction velocity of the electrical signal (dromotropic), and increased rate of relaxation (lusitropic) of cardiac muscle. An increased sympathetic drive increases the myocardial oxygen demand that has to be met by coronary circulation. The coronary blood flow to the left side of the heart is predominantly during the diastole, the duration of which is directly determined by the heart rate. As the heart rate increases, the duration of one beat is reduced, thereby further reducing the duration of diastole, and thus heart rate becomes a major limiting factor. If the heart is diseased, this increase in oxygen demand cannot be met, leading to ischemia. This demand/supply ratio may be affected due to increased sympathetic drive, endothelial damage of the arteries, and an already diseased heart.

High sympathetic drive is seen in postmyocardial infarction cases, and therefore vulnerability to arrhythmias and ischemic events is high in these cases, and they lead to sleep disturbances.

Cardiac arrhythmias are seen during both REM and NREM due to alterations in the sympathetic and parasympathetic drive, as discussed. During NREM, there is a slight reduction in sympathetic drive as compared to being awake and in REM sleep. The reduction in sympathetic drive causes a reduction in volume and velocity of blood flow. During sleep, a prothrombotic milieu prevails, and in the background of vascular endothelial damage, NREM sleep serves as the right time when the reduced blood velocity causes stagnation of blood, and a predilection to the development of thrombi or dislodged emboli exists. Non-demand myocardial infarction during NREM is seen in patients with severe coronary disease, diabetes, and other causes of significant endothelial dysfunction.

EFFECTS OF SLEEP ON THE ENDOCRINE SYSTEM AND METABOLISM

Emerging evidence shows that reduced sleep quality is associated with increased plasma glucose levels, probably due to reduced insulin sensitivity. A reduced slow wave sleep despite similar total sleep time is often reported with reduced sleep quality and is a major determinant of quality apart from many other known and not so known factors. During slow wave sleep, reduced cerebral glucose use is seen, growth hormone secretion increases, the release of cortisol is reduced, and there is a reduced sympathetic and increased parasympathetic drive.

Further, both Process C and Process S determine the sleep propensity, as discussed in Chapters 1 and 2, interact with and modulate the endocrine system, and affect metabolism.

- Hormones affected by sleep-wake or Process S are predominantly growth hormone and prolactin. In normal healthy humans, growth hormone peaks during slow wave sleep at night. Prolactin secretion starts before sleep onset and peaks by the point of midsleep. Various factors can inhibit nocturnal prolactin levels like awakenings, the inhibition of dopamine. Similarly, drugs like benzodiazepines, ramelteon, and zolpidem increase nocturnal prolactin.
- Hormones that are predominantly controlled by circadian rhythm are corticosteroids. It is maximized in the morning and then reduces over the day to reach a minimum. Generally, sleep onset occurs when corticosteroids are at the minimum. Even a partial sleep deprivation causes an evening rise of cortisol the next day.
- Hormones that are affected by both, i.e., both Processes C and S, interact to influence the levels of thyroid-stimulating hormone (TSH). TSH levels are low in the morning, which increase rapidly in the evening. Sleep at night inhibits TSH, but sleep during the afternoon greatly affects the levels, implying both sleep-wake and circadian control on TSH. Night awakenings cause spurts in its levels. Second-night deprivation causes a rise but not as much as the first-night depression.

- The effects of sleep on gonadal axis and reproductive hormones are different in boys and girls.
  - In both prepubertal boys, as well as in girls, luteinising hormone (LH) and follicular stimulating hormone (FSH) are pulsatile. In adults, a pattern emerges and is different in males and in females. In females, the pattern also depends on the phase of menstrual cycle.
  - In males, the day-night differences in LH start to dampen, though LH pulses occur at night related temporally to NREM and REM cycles. In females, during the early follicular phase, there is slowing of frequency of pulses of LH during sleep. In the midfollicular phase, LH pulse amplitude reduces and frequency increases. The effect of sleep on the LH seen in the early follicular phase is less. In the early luteal phase, pulse amplitude increases, and frequency is reduced with nocturnal slowing. In mid- and late luteal phases, pulse amplitude and frequency are both reduced, and the effect of sleep is not seen. LH pulses, awakenings at night, and correlation to REM sleep or NREM sleep has recently generated interest because of changes found in patients of polycystic ovarian disease. It is difficult, however, to ascertain whether it is the cause or the effect of this interaction, but further studies in patients and normal controls might help us understand it better and might provide therapeutic potential for disorders.
  - Postmenopausal women show an increased LH and FSH, but no circadian pattern is seen. Estrogen replacement is documented to improve sleep quality in these patients, especially when they have sleep disordered breathing. The exact mechanism is still unclear.
  - In adult males, testosterone levels are low in evenings. They start rising with the onset of sleep. A rise in the levels is also found during daytime sleep. Hence, sleep deprivation and androgen concentrations in adults may be inversely related.
  - In older men, both LH amplitude and frequency are reduced. There is a dampening

of the circadian variation of testosterone. A sleep-related increase is seen, though the effect is slightly reduced. This effect is also seen in obstructive sleep apnea (OSA) patients.

Sleep and appetite also show an interesting interaction.

- Despite being in a fasting state when asleep overnight, plasma glucose concentrations are very stable, unlike a waking fasted state where a reduction in plasma glucose concentrations is observed. Wake-promoting orexin neurons stimulate food intake. The activity of orexin neurons is inhibited by leptin and stimulated by ghrelin, which are the satiety- and appetite-promoting hormones, respectively. This information is relevant to understand the effects on plasma glucose due to sleep deprivation. Sleep deprivation is known to cause impaired glucose tolerance, reduced insulin sensitivity, and reduction in acute insulin response to glucose, subjecting the individual to an increased risk of diabetes.
- Disorders showing metabolic alterations have effects on sleep. For example, increased levels of proinflammatory cytokines from visceral fat are proposed to cause excessive daytime sleepiness, sleep fragmentation, and fatigue in obese individuals even without OSA. Patients diagnosed with OSA are associated with increased insulin resistance and impaired glucose tolerance. In insomniacs, higher cortisol levels are found during the night. Whether it is the cause of reduced total sleep time or effect is not clear, but an association is clearly and repeatedly reported.

EFFECTS ON NEUROLOGICAL PROCESSING

Memory consolidation is known to occur during sleep. Various experiments show that during NREM, the declarative memory, and during REM, nondeclarative memory are consolidated. Studies also report a relative slowing of sensory and motor processing during sleep. Blood flow to various regions of the brain increases during REM sleep compared to NREM sleep, and there is a differential gradient between regions.

OTHER EFFECTS

Sleep is known to protect the action of natural killer cells. During sleep loss, a reduction in host defense is demonstrated due to multiple direct and indirect effects that are still not clearly elucidated. Systemic inflammation causes acute phase reaction, mediators of which promote sleep. There appears that sleep has some effect on immunity, though the exact mechanisms are still not very evident.

Body temperature regulation during NREM sleep is set at a lower value, and during REM, body temperature tends to drift toward environmental pressures. Penile erections are seen during REM sleep. Erectile dysfunction can be evaluated using penile tumescence, and it can be used to differentiate between a psychological or a pathophysiological cause.

APPLICATIONS OF RECORDING PHYSIOLOGICAL PARAMETERS DURING SLEEP

- Monitoring of sleep can be done better once one knows the normal changes and, if an abnormality appears, what they imply.
- The monitoring of sleep and its disorders can be further enhanced by using specific equipment to clinch the diagnosis.
- ECG recording and pulse plethysmograph signal can be integrated to derive the pulse transit time (PTT), which is the time taken for the arterial pulse wave from the aortic valve to the periphery. It can be calculated by the time between the R-wave and the arrival of the pulse waveform at the finger. PTT can be used to determine noninvasive blood pressure.
- Heart rate variability can be studied using time domain and frequency domain analysis of beat-to-beat R-R intervals data. These spectral transforms predict the predominance of parasympathetic and sympathetic predominance of the body. Though the derivation of these analyses is beyond the scope of this book, but at a concept level, a commonly used method is the frequency domain analysis of ECG signal and the determination of low-frequency (LF), high-frequency (HF) components and their ratio, LF/HF ratio. Increased LF and LF/HF ratio

show a sympathetic predominance, and an increased HF and reduction in LF/HF signify parasympathetic predominance.

- Continuous glucose monitoring at night done for diabetic management relies on the effects of sleep on glucose metabolism and plasma glucose levels during sleep at night.
- The analysis of rate and rhythm from the ECG signal can help identify arrythmias, ischemia, etc.
- Sleep-related bruxism or abnormal movements can be picked up by EMG electrodes on the submentalis muscle and on the limb, respectively.
- Pulse oximetry correlated with respiratory effort and oronasal flow simultaneously can help differentiate different apnea and hypopneas.
- Analysis of bruxism EEG spectrum can help derive microarousals during sleep, which may be further analyzed to correlate their presentation with a respiratory event, desaturations due to respiratory or cardiovascular abnormality, abnormal movements recorded from limb electrodes, or a spontaneous type seen in insomnia.

- In the case of a suspicion of seizure at night, an extended EEG montage may be put in polysomnography to pick up the seizure activity and location.
- Recent advances have been made in the evaluation of sleep disorders: placing transcutaneous CO_2 sensors, transesophageal pressure monitoring, upper GI monitoring for reflux, upper airway MRI to estimate oropharyngeal space, etc.

CONCLUSION

Sleep manifests various physiological changes during sleep. Knowing about them opens up the mind of the practitioner not only in analyzing the sleep study report better but also in picking up clinical signs of impending disease faster.

SUGGESTED READING

1. Barrett KE, Boitano S, Barman SM, Brooks HL, Ganong WF, editors. *Ganong's Review of Medical Physiology*. 25th ed. New York, NY: McGraw-Hill; 2015. 768 p. (A Lange medical book).

4

Respiratory Physiology: Simple Science of CPAP and PAP Devices Explained

DEEPAK SHRIVASTAVA, AND AJITPAL SETHI

DOI: 10.1201/9781003093381-5

RESPIRATORY CHANGES DURING SLEEP

Respiratory changes that occur during sleep are dependent on the staging of the sleep, take place during rapid eye movement sleep versus non rapid eye movement sleep. During sleep, the wakeful drive to breathe goes away and only the metabolic drive initiates ventilation. Central sleep apneas are commonly observed at sleep onset. Upper airway muscle tone is decreased, and there is increased resistance to the airflow. From wakefulness to non-REM sleep, resistance increases and then further increases to the highest level during REM sleep. Because of the reduced tidal volumes, the minute ventilation decreases, as does alveolar ventilation. In sleep, the functional residual capacity declines. Breathing is observed to be regular during non-REM sleep, but it becomes irregular during REM sleep. In wakefulness, both high CO_2 and low PO_2 increase the ventilation. These responses are dampened during sleep. Oxygen concentration in the blood, as well as the oxygen saturation, decreases slightly; however, total oxygen consumption and the production of carbon dioxide are decreased accordingly. In non-REM sleep as well as in REM sleep, cough reflexes are diminished.

Breathing Pattern during Non-REM Sleep

- More regular respiratory pattern than in wakeful breathing
- Reduction in the tidal volume
- Slight rise in CO_2 by 1–2 mmHg

Breathing Pattern during REM Sleep

- Irregular and variable respiratory pattern
- Increased frequency of breathing and reduced tidal volume compared to non-REM sleep
- Further CO_2 increase by 1–2 mmHg
- Oxygen saturation drop at the onset of REM sleep
- Ventilatory responses to high CO_2 and low O_2 differences between REM and non-REM sleep; also variable between men and women
- Possible arousal from sleep triggered by both low oxygen and high CO_2

Response of the Upper Airway Muscles to Sleep

- Upper airway muscles maintain the patency of the upper airways during inspiration and prevent collapse.
- The genioglossus muscle (tongue) responds to the increase in high CO_2 during wakefulness.
- This response is decreased during sleep.
- In normal individuals, the negative pressure reflex during inspiration activates the pharyngeal dilator muscles to keep the airway open. However, at sleep onset and non-REM sleep, this response is significantly reduced. (It can precipitate episodes of apnea or hypopnea by decreasing the effective lumen of the upper airway.)

Effect of the Positional Changes during Sleep

- The supine position can cause narrowing of the upper airway behind the tongue and can predispose to upper airway collapse.
- In the supine position, the functional residual capacity is reduced as increased abdominal distention and viscera push the diaphragm up.
- REM sleep is associated with relative hypoventilation from both reduced ventilatory mechanical capacities and decrease sensitivity of the respiratory drive to high CO_2 and low oxygenation.

RESPIRATORY PHYSIOLOGY IN SLEEP DISORDERED BREATHING

- Narrowing of the upper airway and excess body weight increase the mechanical load on the respiratory system and therefore increase the work of breathing.
- Sleep can perpetuate repetitive events of apneas or hypopneas due to oxygen desaturation.
- Hypopneas are more common during REM sleep.
- Oxygen desaturation is frequent and sustained during REM sleep.
- High CO_2 levels can occur especially in the supine sleep position.

SCIENCE OF CONTINUOUS POSITIVE AIRWAY PRESSURE IN SLEEP DISORDERED BREATHING

Continuous positive airway therapy and its advanced modifications are considered the first-line and most efficacious treatment for sleep disordered breathing. The continuous positive airway pressure increases the oropharyngeal volume and reduces the collapsibility of the pharynx by providing a pneumatic splint. CPAP therapy is titrated to alleviate all apneas, hypopneas, and respiratory-effort-related arousals and reestablishes oxygen saturation to its normal range.

EFFECTIVENESS OF CPAP

A properly titrated continuous positive airway pressure (CPAP) eliminates sleep disordered breathing in most patients. As previously noted, it eliminates snoring, apneas, and hypopneas, as well as reestablishes oxygen saturation to the normal range. CPAP improves the symptoms of daytime sleepiness, as well as cognitive function and mood in patients with mild to moderate sleep disordered breathing. Patients who have concomitant hypertension tend to benefit from CPAP. Although the effect size is limited to a 2–3 mmHg reduction in blood pressure, it has been shown to be more efficacious in lowering blood pressure in patients with severe sleep apnea. For patients who suffer with congestive heart failure with low ejection fraction, CPAP tends to improve the ejection fraction in the subset of the population. CPAP works synergistically with antihypertensive therapy, improves quality of life, and reduces cardiovascular, neurocognitive, and metabolic complications.

Positive airway pressure is a mode of respiratory ventilation that is considered the mainstay treatment of obstructive sleep apnea. CPAP provides a pneumatic splint to maintain upper airway patency during sleep. It prevents the soft tissue from collapsing and prevents partial or complete obstruction of the airway. This results in a decreased number of arousals from sleep and stabilizes oxygen desaturation. In addition, CPAP lowers transmural pressure within the chest cavity, thereby favorably affecting cardiac function.

DATA CARD (SMART CARD OR SD CARD)

Basic CPAP machines blow air to create a pneumatic splint to keep the collapsible part of the airway patent. Some features record CPAP usage by means of a digital smart card. The only things that distinguish all the models are the features that may be available. Of the different manufacturers, some provide unique features than others.

Either CPAP machines are equipped with the SD data card, or a data card can be attached as a separate piece of equipment. The SD data card records the functioning of the machine, indirectly reflecting the usage time, and produces a report over time range to reflect compliance with the treatment. It also reports the residual AHI, the leak percentage, and a range of pressures applied throughout the duration of therapy. Data card information is also very helpful in troubleshooting as it highlights the issues related to the noncompliance of CPAP use due to intolerance and side effects. Certain insurance companies and third-party payers, as well as the department of transportation, uses data card information to establish compliance with the requirements of CPAP use in patients with sensitive occupations like truck drivers or pilots.

POSITIVE AIRWAY PRESSURE DELIVERY: TYPES OF POSITIVE AIRWAY PRESSURE MACHINES AND THEIR UNIQUE FEATURES

A variety of positive airway pressure systems, including continuous positive airway pressure (CPAP), bilevel positive airway pressure (BiPAP), automatic positive airway pressure (APAP), have different user-friendly pressure settings to deliver the positive pressure to the narrowed or obstructed airway in order to increase its patency for normal breathing. Providers may start by utilizing the more common features that patients may or may not need to make usage precise and increase compliance with CPAP use.

PAP therapy increases positive intrathoracic pressure, resulting in decreased venous return, increased lung volume, decreased afterload, and possible increase in cardiac output. Since the pressure is maintained during exhalation, it increases end-expiratory lung volume. Such a traction effect can further assist in the splinting open of the upper airway

Altitude Adjustment

This feature is available on some basic machines but not on others. This may be a useful feature for people living or stationed at high altitude, for example, military personnel, and for those who travel to altitudes often. Altitude adjustments can be either manual or automatic. If one travels once a year to the mountains, manual adjustment may be better; otherwise, auto adjustment may be the better choice.

Ramp Feature

The ramp feature is designed for patient comfort and improved tolerance of the higher levels of pressures. The CPAP starts at lower pressure and, coincident with the patient's drowsiness and falling asleep, the pressure rises slowly to the desired prescribed pressure. Most ramp features allow 15 minutes of ramp time, which can be reset by the push of the ramp button on the CPAP machine.

Auto-CPAP machines generally start with 4–5 cm of water pressure and gradually adjust the pressure to the patient's requirement, based on the subtle feedback mechanism that responds to the airflow or pressure changes, until the pressure rises to optimal flow. The ramp feature should be recommended to most patients in order to increase their level of comfort and tolerance that translates into better compliance with CPAP use.

EPR (Expiratory Pressure Relief): ResMed and C-Flex or Bi-Flex

Studies have shown that CPAP or BIPAP compliance is better when using the EPR (expiratory pressure relief), C-Flex, or Bi-Flex features. Currently, there are only two major manufacturers of this technology: ResMed (EPR) and Respironics (C-Flex or Bi-Flex). As of this writing, no other major manufacturers provide this feature.

An easy way to explain these features is that it is harder to breathe against fast airflow. The greater the airflow, the harder it can be to breathe. The same principle applies to CPAP machines when they blow air. Most people can tolerate about 7–8 cm of water pressure and can breathe against it. EPR and C-Flex/Bi-Flex respond to each breath throughout the night and provide relief. *This feature gives the device the ability to make breath-by-breath adjustments to*

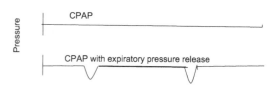

Figure 4.1 CPAP with expiratory pressure release

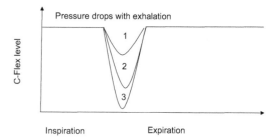

Figure 4.2 C-Flex pressure drops with exhalation (3- settings)

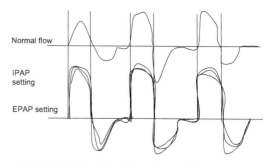

Choice of three Bi-Flex settings for transition comfort

Figure 4.3 Bi-Flex pressure changes during both inhalation and exhalation (3-settings)

ensure the optimal level of pressure relief during exhalation in order to deliver more comfortable therapy.

Humidification

Humidity helps to open and keep the interior of the nasal passages open. The drying action of the air without humidity tends to make the airway more restricted in many situations.

BASIC FUNCTIONING OF POSITIVE AIRWAY PRESSURE MACHINES

CPAP eliminates snoring sounds by opening up the airway. CPAP maintains the same pressure during the inspiratory phase as well as the expiratory phase of the respiratory cycle.

Bilevel pressure devices (BiPAP) are different from CPAP only in that they deliver higher inspiratory positive pressure and lower expiratory positive pressure for easier exhalation. BiPAP pressure can be delivered in different modes:

S (spontaneous) mode: The device triggers inspiratory pressure when flow sensors detect spontaneous respiratory effort.

T (timed) mode: The inspiratory-to-expiratory cycling is machine triggered at a set rate and timed to a certain number of breaths per minute.

S/T (spontaneous/timed): A BiPAP machine triggers the inspiratory pressure response in response to the patient's inspiratory effort. However, the S/T mode provides a backup rate to provide a minimum number of breaths if a patient is unable to take spontaneous breaths.

CONTINUOUS POSITIVE AIRWAY PRESSURE (CPAP)

CPAP remains the mainstay of therapy for obstructive sleep apnea syndrome (OSAS). CPAP therapy has been demonstrated to resolve sleep disordered breathing events and improve several clinical outcomes. CPAP is conventionally delivered via a nasal mask at a fixed pressure that remains constant throughout the respiratory cycle. CPAP therapy exerts its beneficial effects by acting as a pneumatic splint to prevent the upper airway soft tissue from collapsing.

Indications for CPAP therapy include:

- Treatment of moderate to severe OSAS.
- Treatment of mild OSAS and associated symptoms and/or underlying cardiovascular disease.

AUTOMATIC CPAP (APAP)

Automatic CPAP (APAP) is also known as auto-, automated, auto adjusting, or auto titrating continuous positive airway pressure.

APAP further advances CPAP therapy with the ability to detect and respond to changes in upper airway resistance in real time. APAP noninvasively detects variations of upper airway obstruction and airflow limitation, including snoring, hypopneas, and apneas. The sensors used to detect the spectrum of an upper airway obstruction, such as detecting snoring via a mask, vary among APAP models. Once upper airway flow limitation has been detected, the APAP device automatically increases the pressure until the flow limitation has been resolved. Once a therapeutic pressure has been achieved, the APAP device reduces pressure until flow limitation resumes.

BILEVEL POSITIVE PRESSURE THERAPY (BIPAP)

As opposed to CPAP therapy, which allows a fixed pressure throughout the respiratory cycle, bilevel therapy allows the independent adjustment of the expiratory and inspiratory positive airway pressures (PAP). Bilevel therapy remains a viable option for CPAP-intolerant patients who have OSAS, OSAS with concurrent respiratory disease, and/or obesity hypoventilation syndrome. BiPAP or VPAP machines are, in many cases, prescribed by the physician if patients cannot tolerate CPAP during the sleep study or have trouble tolerating higher pressures.

In a nutshell, a BiPAP machine basically has two pressures: an inspiratory pressure, which is the pressure of the blowing air during inhalation, and an expiratory pressure, which is typically reduced during exhalation. It is designed to provide relief if the patient is unable to tolerate higher pressures.

Normal breathing, without the use of any equipment, is negative pressure breathing (breathing at atmospheric pressure). Equipment like CPAP is used to splint the airway with positive pressure or PAP (positive airway pressure), which is higher than atmospheric pressure:

IPAP: Inspiratory positive airway pressure—measured in cmH_2O
EPAP: Expiratory positive airway pressure—measured in cmH_2O

- BiPAP alternates between IPAP and EPAP and synchronizes with the patient's breathing.
- Normal respiration has two phases, inspiration and expiration, plus a pause between them.

- BiPAP aids during the inspiratory phase and prevents airway closure during the expiratory phase.
- The normal inspiratory-to-expiratory ratio (I:E ratio) is 1:2.
- As the patient inspires, the BiPAP delivers IPAP, which stops as the patient expires, but pressure within the airway remains positive because of EPAP.
- BiPAP delivers CPAP but also senses when inspiratory effort is being made and delivers a higher pressure during inspiration.
- When inspiration plus IPAP stop, pressure returns to the EPAP level.

AVAPS (AVERAGE VOLUME ASSURED PRESSURE SUPPORT)

- AVAPS is a mode that is added to S mode, S/T mode, or T mode.
- AVAPS can be used with or without the backup rate.
- AVAPS takes away the need to titrate IPAP but still needs to titrate EPAP.
- BiPAP S/T with AVAPS is designed to deliver a set tidal volume (VT) to patients with respiratory insufficiency.
- The S/T with AVAPS feature provides three types of support to patients:
  - Pressure to the airway to prevent airway collapse
  - Backup rate for patients who encounter central apneas
  - Automatically adjusting pressure support that ensures the set tidal volume
- AVAPS is designed to maintain a target VT the entire night.
- AVAPS maintains VT for long-term use as the disease progresses.
- AVAPS uses pressure to maintain the set VT.
- The pressure that ensures the VT is dependent on:
  - Patient effort.
  - Lung compliance.
  - Airway resistance.
- If the set VT is not delivered, the pressure is gradually increased to deliver the set VT.
- If the VT exceeds the set VT, the pressure is gradually decreased.

BIPAP S/T WITH AVAPS: TITRATION

- Settings for S/T with AVAPS:

> Rate
> Rise time
> EPAP
> I time
> IPAP min = minimum inspiratory pressure
> IPAP max = maximum inspiratory pressure
> Tidal volume

The set tidal volume is based on:

- Patient breathing on the system for 4 minutes: 110% of the average displayed *or* the patient's ideal body weight (8 mg/kg of ideal) for height and gender.
- Don't forget patient comfort: adjust the VT for patient comfort and tolerance.

Recommended Starting Points

- Starting in S/T mode with AVAPS on
- EPAP at 4 cmH$_2$O
- IPAP min 8 cmH$_2$O (adjusted up or down based on patient comfort)
- Set tidal volume (per the preceding recommendations)
- IPAP max (initially not "wide open"—you can always adjust upward)
- Rate of 8–10 BPM or 2 BPM below the patient's spontaneous rate
- I-time of 1.2 (adjust based on patient comfort and preceding recommendations)
- Rise time at 2–3

S/T with AVAPS maintains the tidal volume by slowly increasing or decreasing the pressure.
AVAPS uses pressure to maintain the set tidal volume throughout the night.

S/T AVAPS Indications

Patients with:

- Neuromuscular disease
- Chronic obstructive pulmonary disease
- Obesity hypoventilation syndrome

Note

- The automatic algorithm changes based on patient needs.
- Slow adjustment over time takes 1 minute for each increase.

BIPAP AVAPS (AVERAGE VOLUME ASSURED PRESSURE SUPPORT)

BiPAP AVAPS (average volume assured pressure support) is designed to maintain tidal volumes for patients who have respiratory insufficiency and who need noninvasive ventilator support.

BiPAP AVAPS provides three types of support:

- A backup rate to assist patients who have difficulty maintaining a consistent respiratory rate.
- Pressure support to assist patients who have difficulty maintaining tidal volume.
- Expiratory pressure to assist patients who need to increase their FRC (functional residual capacity) or maintain airway stability.

Indications

- Restrictive disorders—kyphosis, fibrosis
- Neuromuscular disorders
- OSAS
- Obesity hypoventilation syndrome
- COPD
- Periodic breathing—rarely used
- Complex sleep apnea—rarely used

The indications are the same as for BiPAP Auto SV. While one can technically use Auto SV in NMD patients, S/T with AVAPS is preferred.

Settings for BiPAP AVAPS

- Rate
- Rise time
- EPAP pressure
- Inspiratory time
- Tidal volume
- IPAP minimum
- IPAP maximum

AVAPS IS *NOT* RECOMMENDED FOR PERIODIC BREATHING SUCH AS CHEYNE–STOKES

AVAPS does not respond fast enough. The event would be over before the needed pressure is reached, i.e., the length of the event vs. the time of response are mismatched. The solution for such patient would be AutoSV (see the next module).

AUTOSV: *NOT* RECOMMENDED FOR NEUROMUSCULAR DISEASE

- AutoSV would continually reset its baseline and increase hypoventilation.
- The normal target would continue to decrease and continue to under ventilate the patient as the night progresses.

The solution for this NMD patient or a patient with obesity hypoventilation syndrome is AVAPS.

- AVAPS maintains the set VT.
- AVAPS has a slow reaction (0.5–1.0 cmH$_2$O increase over 1 minute).

The BMI is the parameter that is *not* considered when determining the target VT with AVAPS.

PRIMARY CARE MANAGEMENT OF POSITIVE AIRWAY PRESSURE THERAPY

The understanding of the function of the airway, as well as the pathophysiology of the narrowing of the airway by collapse, is further confounded by factors like obesity, craniofacial abnormalities, soft tissue abnormalities, bony abnormalities, and functional abnormalities of the upper airway. The primary care provider can, however, explain the mechanism of airway obstruction to patients and prepare them for what to expect after the diagnosis is made and how treatment will help their condition.

Once the patient begins to use CPAP, the primary care provider is generally the first resource for troubleshooting. A working knowledge of the respiratory physiology of positive airway pressure is useful in understanding how the patient's reported problems may cause intolerance and noncompliance with CPAP use.

This knowledge empowers the primary care physician to make a clinical decision for referral to the sleep specialist for providing intervention and assistance.

SUGGESTED READING

1. Antonescu-Turcu A, Parthasarathy S. CPAP and bi-level PAP therapy: new and established roles. *Respir Care*. 2010;55(9):1216–1229.
2. Bakker J, Marshall N. *Chest*. 2011;139:1322–1330.
3. Ballard D, et al. *J Clin Sleep Med*. 2007;3:706–712.
4. Murphy P, et al. *Thorax*. 2012;67:727–734.

5

Drugs That Affect Sleep

DEEPAK SHRIVASTAVA

Sleep is organized into two stages known as non-rapid eye movement (NREM) sleep and rapid eye movement (REM) sleep. These stages are identifiable by specific parameters and have characteristic patterns. Sleep stages are affected by pharmaceuticals in nearly every drug category. This chapter reviews the effect of medications on sleep architecture and their clinical significance.

In the wakeful state of the brain, the EEG shows low voltage and fast frequency of 10–30 μV and 16–26 Hz, respectively. In stage N1 non-REM sleep, the EEG slows down to 3–7 Hz and decreases in amplitude. Stage N2 non-REM sleep is characterized by the appearance of sleep spindles (12–14 Hz) and K-complexes. Stage N3 non-REM sleep is also known as slow wave sleep or delta sleep; the EEG shows 0.5–2 Hz waves of 75 μV or greater. In REM sleep, the EEG shows a low-voltage, mixed-frequency pattern similar to stage 1 non-REM sleep. However, the electro-oculogram of REM sleep shows bursts of rapid eye movements, and the electromyogram (EMG) shows a complete atonia of the muscles.

While adults enter sleep through stage I, non-REM and REM sleep cycle 4–5 times per night, and each cycle is approximately 90 minutes. The percentage of non-REM vs. REM sleep changes over the night, and REM sleep is longer during the second half of the night. In general, total sleep time is divided into 5% of N1, 50% N2, 20% N3, and 25% REM sleep, also known as stage R.

SEROTONERGIC ANTAGONIST

Drugs like ritanserin increase stage N3 but generally do not improve sleep time or insomnia-related symptoms. Another related drug, ketanserin, reduces the number of awakenings and wake after sleep onset time compared to ritanserin.

DOI: 10.1201/9781003093381-6

EFFECT OF MEDICATION ON SLEEP

Sleep architecture and quality can be affected by any medications that cross the blood–brain barrier. Sleep quality can be defined as a restorative sleep that makes someone feel refreshed upon awakening in the morning and able to maintain alertness and wakefulness throughout the day.

The architecture of sleep is how sleep is structured, and it cycles between non-rapid eye movement and rapid eye movement sleep approximately 4–5 times on an average night. Sleep quality can be measured by subjective feelings as well as objectively by how long it takes to fall asleep, how many times someone wakes up after falling asleep, and the amount of sleep in terms total hours.

Medications can affect sleep in both a positive and a negative manner. Some factors are therapeutic and can be used to induce and maintain good-quality sleep; on the other hand, some medications cause sleep interruption, lightened stages of sleep, and sleep fragmentation, causing tiredness during the daytime. Medications can also decrease or increase sleep architecture and quality, as well as the amount of sleep in different stages.

Many medications include benzodiazepines, Z-drugs, antiepileptic medications, antidepressants, stimulants, and analgesics, along with various cardiac and pulmonary medications

BENZODIAZEPINE'S EFFECT ON SLEEP

BENZODIAZEPINE RECEPTOR AGONISTS

This class of drug includes benzodiazepines and nonbenzodiazepine medications. Benzodiazepines reduce stage N3 sleep. Triazolam does not appear to have any effect on the sleep stages, nor is it a means to increase total sleep time and quality of self-reported sleep.

These drugs are represented by lorazepam, midazolam, and diazepam, medications used to treat anxiety and insomnia. These medications work through GABA receptors, which are present throughout the brain.

Benzodiazepines cause significant changes in sleep architecture. The overall effect is reducing sleep easily, reducing the nighttime awakenings, and increasing total sleep time. During the day, individuals experience less sleepiness and better concentration with a decreasing level of alertness throughout the day. Their discontinuation can cause rebound insomnia.

Table 5.1 shows the effects of barbiturates, benzodiazepines, and nonbenzodiazepine medications on various sleep parameters.

1. Benzodiazepines reduce the amount of N1 sleep.

Table 5.1 Benzodiazepines vs. Barbiturates.

Parameter	Barbiturate	BZD	Non-BZD
TST (total sleep time)	⇧⇧⇧	⇧⇧⇧	⇧⇧
Sleep latency	⇩⇩⇩	⇩⇩⇩	⇩⇩⇩
N2 sleep	⇧⇧	⇧⇧	⇔
N3 sleep	⇩	⇩⇩	⇔
REM sleep	⇩⇩⇩	⇩	⇔
Withdrawal	Adverse events	Rebound insomnia	Minor
Overdose risk	High	Low	Low

2. They increase spindle density and activity during N2 sleep and increase the amount of N2 sleep.
3. They may reduce REM sleep in high doses.

Clinical Implications

- Daytime sedation with long-acting agents
- Short acting agents: rebound insomnia
- May worsen OSA
- Rapid withdrawal: nightmares/arousals
- Suppression of N3 sleep: nonrestorative sleep

Z-DRUGS (NONBENZODIAZEPINE RECEPTOR AGONISTS)

The nonbenzodiazepine medications do not tend to have a significant effect on sleep architecture but do improve sleep efficiency and total sleep time. In clinical doses, these drugs do not suppress REM sleep.

Drugs like gamma hydroxybutyrate and sodium salt of GHB sodium oxybate are GABA-B agonists. They increase the increased percentage of slow wave sleep but have no impact on total sleep time. These medications are generally used in the treatment of narcolepsy.

- Z-drugs reduce the amount of N1 sleep, which is considered a drowsy state, and therefore these medications have therapeutic effect/
- They also increase spinal activity during N2 sleep with an increased percentage of N2 sleep.
- They have variable effects on slow wave sleep.
- The stress may modestly reduce REM sleep, and high doses may increase their overall risk.

Sedative-hypnotic drug products (benzodiazepines and nonbenzodiazepines) can cause:

- Increase incidents of sleepwalking.
- Automatic driving without the awareness of location and how the distance was covered.
- Eating during sleep without any knowledge or recollection of the event with unexplained weight gain.

OREXIN RECEPTOR ANTAGONISTS

Recently, the new medications Lemborexant and suvorexant were approved by the FDA for the treatment of insomnia. These medications cause a profound effect on the maintenance of sleep compared to sleep induction at bedtime. As a side effect, these medications can cause impaired driving performance.

1. Suvorexant improves sleep onset and maintains sleep throughout the night, improving sleep quality.
2. The increased REM pressure can cause increased duration of REM sleep and REM density and reduce the REM latency.
3. Other sleep stages in non-REM sleep are unaffected.

MELATONIN

Ramelteon is a melatonin receptor agonist. Melatonin and melatonin receptor agonists are generally prescribed for the treatment of sleep onset insomnia. Tasimelteon has recently been approved as a probiotic for the treatment of circadian rhythm sleep disorders and non-24-hour sleep-wake disorder. Individuals do not consistently experience increased total sleep duration or improvement in the daytime functioning. These medications do improve the ability to fall asleep.

- These medications reduce the latency to sleep onset and increase sleep duration, thereby improving the quality of the sleep.
- There are inconsistent effects on sleep maintenance.
- Ramelteon reduces the amount of N1 sleep, which is considered a good therapeutic effect.
- Melatonin's effect on sleep architecture is inconsistent.

NEWER NON-D2 NEUROLEPTICS

The newer non-D2 neuroleptics are clozapine, olanzapine, risperidone (chlorpromazine, haloperidol, thioridazine).

- Increased sedation: daytime sleepiness
- Decreased N3: nonrestorative sleep
- Increased RLS and PLMD: sleep fragmentation

Table 5.2 shows the effect of the adrenergic medications on sleep parameters.

Table 5.2 Adrenergic and Sleep (REM = rapid eye movement sleep; NE = norepinephrine).

Drug	Action	Effect
Phenylephrine	Alpha 1 agonist	↑ Arousal
Clonidine	Alpha 2 agonist	↑ Sedation
Prazosin	Alpha 1 agonist	↑ REM ↓ Nightmare
Yohimbine	Alpha 2 agonist	↑ Wake
Mirtazapine/Remeron	Alpha 2 agonist	↑ Sedation
Propranolol	B blocker	↑ Wake, nightmare
Reserpine	NE store depletion	↑ REM

DOPAMINE AND NE EFFECTIVE STIMULANTS

Dopamine and NE effective stimulants include:

- Pemoline (Cylert).
- Mazindol (Sanorex).
- Selegiline (Eldepry).
- Amphetamine (Adderall).
- *D*-amphetamine (Dexedrine).
- *L*-amphetamine.
- Methamphetamine (Desoxyn).
- Methylphenidate (Ritalin).
- Cocaine (DA and NE reuptake inhibitor).
- Ecstasy (DA and NE reuptake inhibitor).

Dopamine and NE effective stimulants increase wakefulness, wakefulness after sleep onset (WASO), and RLS and decrease total sleep time (TST), REM, and N3 sleep.

- Table 5.3 shows medications that work on sleep parameters through the serotonin neuromodulator effect.
- Table 5.4 shows generally used SSRI medications and their effect on stages of sleep, as well as the inability to cause sedation. Both generic and commercial names are provided.

- Table 5.5 shows typical tricyclic antidepressant medications and their effects on sleep stages as well as sedation. Amitriptyline, doxepin, and trimipramine tend to be more sedating, while clomipramine suppresses REM sleep significantly.
- Table 5.6 shows some antidepressant medications and their modes of action. The effects on different sleep stages are displayed.

ANTIEPILEPTICS: EFFECT ON SLEEP

These drugs include phenobarbital, carbamazepine, and phenytoin. The newer drugs include gabapentin, tiagabine, and pregabalin. Levetiracetam is also a new antiseizure drug.

Levetiracetam can potentially increase daytime sleepiness if taken at high doses.

1. The older drugs like phenobarbital have variable effects on sleep architecture. Phenobarbital decreases REM sleep.
2. Carbamazepine can increase stage N3 sleep and reduce stage R (REM).
3. Dilantin increases stage N1 and reduces stage N3.
4. The newer antiseizure drugs increase the patient's tendency to sleep and reduces REM sleep.

Table 5.3 Serotonin and Sleep (REM density = rapid eye movements; SL= sleep latency; SSRI= selective serotonin reuptake inhibitor).

Drug	Action	Effect
Tryptophan	Precursor	↑ N3, REM density, SL
LSD-25	Antagonist	↑ REM, REMs in N3
Buspirone	Antagonist	No effect
Cyproheptadine	Antagonist	↑ N3
SSRI	Agonist	↓ N3, REM, sedation

Table 5.4 *Selective* Serotonin Reuptake Inhibitor.

Drug	N3	Rem	Sedation
Fluoxetine PROZAC	=/↓	=/↓	↓
Paroxetine PAXIL	=/↓	↓↓	↓↓
Sertraline ZOLOFT	=	↓↓	=

Table 5.5 Tricyclic Antidepressants and Sleep.

Drug	N3	REM	Sedation
Amitriptyline	↑	↓↓↓	↑↑↑↑
Doxepin	↑↑	↓↓	↑↑↑↑
Trimipramine	↑	=	↑↑↑↑
Imipramine	↑	↓↓	↑↑
Nortriptyline	↑	↓↓	↑↑
Desipramine	↑	↓↓	↑
Clomipramine	↑	↓↓↓↓	↓/↓

Table 5.6 Antidepressants and Antimanic (DA= dopamine; NA= noradrenaline; 5-HT= hydroxy tryptamine or serotonin).

Drug	Action	Effect
Bupropion	DA and NA modulators	⬆ REM
Nefazodone	5HT antagonist and NE reuptake inhibitor	⬆ REM
Trazodone	Adrenoceptor antagonist and 5HT reuptake inhibitor	⬆ N3 and ⬇ REM
Lithium	—	⬆ REM and ⬇ N3

Alpha-2 Delta Ligand's (Antiepileptic Drugs)

Pregabalin increases stage N3 sleep and reduces the number of awakenings. Another alpha-2 delta acting drug, gabapentin, is used for seizures and neuropathic pain. Gabapentin increases the percentage of N3 sleep but does not change the sleep stages.

ANTIDEPRESSANTS

These medications include tricyclic agents, MAO (monoamine oxidase) inhibitors, selective serotonin reuptake inhibitors (SSRIs), and serotonin antagonist reuptake inhibitors. These medications affect both sleep architecture and sleep quality.

- All antidepressants suppress REM sleep, except that serotonin antagonist may take elevators.
- REM latency is prolonged and is associated with a reduction in the percentage of REM sleep.
- Trazodone increases in stage N3 sleep.
- Desipramine decreases stage N3 sleep.
- SSRIs increase in stage N1 sleep.
- Tricyclic antidepressants (TCAs) like doxepin, amitriptyline, and trimipramine shorten sleep latency and total wakefulness after sleep onset (WASO).
- Nortriptyline and aspirin may have little or no effect on sleep onset or sleep maintenance.
- SSRIs like fluoxetine, paroxetine, and sertraline increase wakefulness after sleep onset and decrease total sleep time.

- Lithium increases total sleep time and may decrease REM sleep and increase slow wave N3 sleep.

REM sleep rebound and sleep disturbance can occur with the abrupt discontinuation of REM–sleep-suppressing antidepressants.

DOPAMINERGIC AGONIST

Dopaminergic agonists include levodopa, pergolide, pramipexole, and prednisone ropinirole.

- Levodopa works by means of unknown mechanisms. However, it may inhibit pedunculopontine nucleus and enhance atonia. Clinically, it may increase or decrease N3 and stage R REM sleep.
- Pergolide is a D1 and D2 receptor agonist. Pergolide increases the total sleep time but decreases N3 sleep.
- Pramipexole is a D3 receptor agonist. It does not change total sleep time or sleep efficiency. However, it increases REM latency and decreases the total amount of REM sleep. It is associated with vivid dreams and hallucinations, as well as sudden sleep attacks without any warning.
- Ropinirole is a D3 and D4 receptor agonist that increases total sleep time, sleep efficiency, and stage shifts. However, it does not have any effect on N3 or REM sleep.

RAMELTEON (ROZEREM)

Ramelteon is a nonscheduled prescription drug that works as an MT 1 and MT 2 receptor agonist.

It does not affect N3 sleep, REM sleep, or sleep continuity. It is nonsedating and a relatively safe drug.

OPIATES AND SLEEP

Opiates have a significant effect on sleep. Opiates can increase wakefulness and the number of stage shifts in the sleep and waking states. Opiates decrease total sleep time (TST), decrease sleep efficiency (SE), decrease N3, and rapid eye movement sleep. Opiates cause daytime sedation and central sleep apneas. The sudden withdrawal of opiates can lead to insomnia and nightmares. In patients with obstructive sleep apnea, opiates can worsen the clinical syndrome of apneas and hypopneas.

HYPOLIPIDEMIA AND ANTIARRHYTHMICS

Drugs in this category include simvastatin and lovastatin, which can cause insomnia in susceptible individuals. A few case reports support this finding.

- **Cholestyramine** causes insomnia in a small subset of the population up to 1.3%.
- **Gemfibrozil** can cause drowsiness according to case reports.
- **Disopyramide** or **quinidine** causes fatigue in approximately 3–10% of subjects.
- **Mexiletine** can cause drowsiness and fatigue in 5–10% of patients.
- **Amiodarone** causes fatigue and insomnia in 5–10% of patients.
- **Diltiazem** causes fatigue in 10% of patients.

ANTIHISTAMINES AND SLEEP

Drugs in this group include cimetidine and ranitidine (H2 antagonist), diphenhydramine, brompheniramine, and triprolidine (all H1 antagonists).

- **Cimetidine** increases N3 sleep.
- **Ranitidine** has no effect on sleep.
- **Diphenhydramine** increases sedation.
- **Triprolidine** and brompheniramine reduce stage R or REM sleep.

Nonsedating antihistamines include fexofenadine and loratadine, and sedating antihistamines include sertraline, chlorpheniramine, clemastine, diphenhydramine, hydroxyzine, promethazine, and trifluridine.

MODAFINIL

Modafinil is a selective GABA inhibitor in the sleep promoting regions of the brain. It increases histaminergic activity in the posterior hypothalamus and inhibits sleep inducing area activity in the anterior hypothalamus. Modafinil in clinical doses does not cause any change in sleep architecture. While it is used for reducing sleepiness in narcolepsy patients, it has greater activity on cataplexy.

OVER-THE-COUNTER MEDICATIONS

An estimated three out of four people routinely self-medicate with over-the-counter medications. At this time, more than 300,000 over-the-counter products are available in the market. Over-the-counter medications have an important role in the quality and amount of sleep.

As previously noted, antihistamines cause sleepiness, while decongestants reduce sleep continuously and reduce insomnia. Common decongestants are oxymetazoline (Afrin, Claritin, and Dristan), pseudoephedrine (Sudafed, Actifed), phenylephrine (Sudafed PE), tetrahydrozoline (Visine), and naphazoline (Clear Eyes). Some decongestants can cause sleepiness.

Cough medications and expectorants may cause sleepiness or insomnia depending on individual sensitivity. Dextromethorphan is a cough suppressant (Benylin DM, Delsym, Robitussin DM, Sucrets, TheraFlu, Triaminic, and Formula 44). Guaifenesin is an expectorant (Mucinex, Duratuss, Altarussin, and Robitussin). Both insomnia and sleepiness are possible with antitussives and expectorants. Insomnia can also be induced with nicotine withdrawal.

RECREATIONAL DRUGS AND SLEEP

Alcohol, nicotine, and caffeine can alter sleep both separately and in combination. Cocaine, methamphetamine, ecstasy, and marijuana have a pronounced effect on sleep. These drugs interfere with the neurotransmission of an increasing number of impulses.

Methamphetamine alters dopamine transmission and causes neurons to fire more, resulting in a euphoric feeling. After the drug wears off, dopamine levels drop, and the user "crashes." Cocaine works in a similar manner. Nicotine increases dopamine release and works similarly to methamphetamine and cocaine. Nicotine effects are concentration dependent and cause mild sedation and relaxation in low nicotine concentration and arousal and agitation with high necrotic concentration due to cholinergic effect on the cholinergic receptors.

Caffeine exerts its effect within 15–30 minutes and has a half-life of 3–7 hours. By blocking the adenosine receptors, it causes the temporary relief of sleepiness. However, caffeine disrupts subsequent sleep with more arousals and reduced periods of REM sleep. Caffeine also exerts a diuretic effect.

Alcohol binds to GABA receptors and amplifies its hyperpolarization effect, causing sedation. The major effects of alcohol include acute transient sedation, hyperarousal after sedation, suppression of upper airway muscles leading to increased snoring and sleep apnea, gastritis and GERD, and polyuria. The effects of alcohol can be documented by many months of poor sleep after abstinence.

HERBAL MEDICATIONS

Many herbal medications are available, like valerian root, chamomile, St. John's wort, rosemary, kava kava, and poppy seeds. These products can induce sedation.

- **Valerian** inhibits GABA receptors and increases REM and N3 sleep. Several small studies are available on the sleep-inducing properties of valerian root.
- **Kava** can cause hepatotoxicity and dermopathy.
- **Chamomile** causes only a slight decrease in sleep latency.

SUGGESTED READING

1. Gardenhire DS. Sleep and sleep pharmacology. In *Rau's Respiratory Care Pharmacology*. 8th ed. Louis, MO: Mosby; 2011. pp. 399–416.
2. Proctor A, Bianchi MT. Clinical pharmacology in sleep medicine. *ISRN Pharmacol.* 2012;2012:914168. http://doi.org/10.5402/2012/914168
3. Kanji S, Mera A, Hutton B, et al. Pharmacological interventions to improve sleep in hospitalized adults: a systematic review. *BMJ Open.* 2016;6:e012108. http://doi.org/10.1136/bmjopen-2016-012108
4. Carter G. The pharmacology of parasomnias and movement disorders of sleep. In *Sleep Medicine and the Evolution of Contemporary Sleep Pharmacotherapy*, edited by Denis Larrivee. London: Intech Open; 2021. http://doi.org/10.5772/intechopen.100472.

PART 2

What Does One Do If the Patient Complains of Sleep Problems?

6

Does the Patient Go to Bed on Time at Night and Can't Sleep?

KARUNA DATTA

INTRODUCTION

Insomnia is widely prevalent and a common symptom among outpatients and hospitalized patients. These patients complain of the inability to sleep after going to bed to sleep. The symptoms may occur transiently associated with some specific reason. This reason may be related to a recent event that acts as a stressor. The stressor in these cases is identifiable, may be at any location such as at home or at the workplace, or may be due to a loss of a near and dear one, spouse, or children. It may also be due to the tension of deadlines that are to be kept at work. A detailed history taking reveals the presence of intermittent insomnia-like symptom that, if unattended, manifests as insomnia disorder. In some patients, it may not show as an intermittent pattern but might just transcend gradually to a full-blown chronic insomnia after a specific identifiable stressor. The presentations may vary, reasons may differ, and hence the approach toward treatment is more individualized. Treatment also is gradual and requires regular follow-ups before finally being fully treated. There may be relapses with a stressor later, but the patient who learns the individualized approach can prevent it from further precipitating into a disorder.

DEFINING INSOMNIA

As per *International Classification of Sleep Disorders*, 3rd edition (*ICSD*-3), a persistent difficulty with the initiation of sleep duration, consolidation, or quality that occurs despite adequate opportunity to sleep and results in daytime impairment is defined as insomnia.

In the case that a daytime impairment or a daytime dysfunction is not present, then it limits itself to being an insomnia symptom but not a disorder. This spectrum of an intermittent symptomatology to an established insomnia disorder may at times take years. A detailed history taking with timeline is necessary to establish this diagnosis.

Daytime symptoms are of significance in the diagnosis of insomnia. Daytime complaints in adults may be prominently physical in nature like headache, palpitations, muscle pain, and fatigue, or they may be psychological in nature like mood alterations, irritability, aggressiveness, and reduced motivation with or without cognitive impairment. These symptoms reduce the quality of life of the patient.

Insomnia may coexist with other comorbid disorders, and in such cases, it should be diagnosed as per the criteria of *ICSD*-3. In cases where

DOI: 10.1201/9781003093381-8

insomnia symptoms are found concomitantly with other medical, psychiatric, and/or other sleep disorders, the diagnosis of insomnia is given only when there is an independence in its onset or progression from other disorders and the insomnia persists even after treatment of the concomitant disorder. In case the symptom of insomnia is resolved with the treatment of the concomitant disorder, then the diagnosis of insomnia is not made.

Depending on the duration of the disease, it may be categorized as acute or short-term and chronic insomnia. Usually, in adults, symptoms of difficulty in the onset of sleep, maintaining sleep, or waking up earlier than the desired time are seen. In children and elderly, resistance to go to bed at bedtime and difficulty sleeping without a parent or caregiver is noticed. If the symptoms last for more than 3 times a week and for more than 3 months, it is called chronic insomnia.

At times, episodes of insomnia complaints are less than 3 months each but are spread out over several years. Though intermittent in nature but due to the long duration of symptoms, the diagnosis of chronic insomnia is recommended as per ICSD-3 guidelines.

Patients on hypnotic medications may have symptoms when they stop the medication. If the symptoms last for more than 3 months, then a diagnosis of chronic insomnia can be given. The criteria for diagnosis of acute insomnia or short-term insomnia disorder are similar to those of chronic insomnia in the sense that there is difficulty initiating sleep, maintaining sleep, or waking up too early with daytime complaints despite having adequate opportunity to sleep and no explanation by another sleep disorder, but the symptoms are present for less than 3 months.

MODELS OF INSOMNIA

The pathophysiology of insomnia is explained using various models. Some of the models with implications from the point of treatment modality for insomnia patients are briefly explained next.

1. **Stimulus control model:** According to this model, a stimulus is paired with a behavior. Once paired with the stimulus, the paired behavior is seen. Thus using this model, therapy can target using a stimulus that can control the onset of sleep due to its pairing with sleep onset. For example, a particular music, if presented with sleep, will produce sleep when presented with the same music. The model is utilized in treatment in the case of insomnia where it is proposed that physically altering the sleep environment may induce sleep.

2. **Spielman 3P model:** The 3P model brings out predisposing, perpetuating, and precipitating factors as factors implicated in the pathogenesis of insomnia.
   - Predisposing factors are the biological, psychological, and social factors, e.g., the personality of the individual, age, alcohol consumption, history of smoking can predispose an individual.
   - Perpetuating factors are those factors that are habits or beliefs of the patients followed by them in a hope to better their sleep. For example, lying in bed for a long time to completely recover the lack of sleep. This sleep extension is a perpetuating factor for insomnia, and treatment hence would focus on restriction of time in bed.
   - Precipitating factors are acute occurrences that can trigger insomnia. These are the events or circumstances that may precipitate the chance of insomnia, e.g., life stressors, divorce, death of a near or dear one, illness in family, etc.

3. **Neurocognitive model:** This model discusses the role of cortical arousal and altered sensory processing responsible for a sleep state misperception that might occur. The model holds that insomniacs develop mesograde amnesia of sleep, which can be treated with hypnotics and might help patients especially in cases of sleep state perception.

4. **Psychobiological inhibition model:** The failure to inhibit wakefulness leads to insomnia probably due to the hypersecretion of orexin. Orexin antagonists have been tried as a treatment strategy based on this model.

5. **Cage exchange model:** In a stress response in more of a social context, the sleep pattern becomes a sleep-wake intermediate state.

6. **Drosophila model:** This model holds that there is a genetic component to insomnia

in providing sleep opportunity and may be important for diagnostics and the genetic basis of treatment in future.

MANAGING INSOMNIA

1. **Ascertaining the diagnosis:**
   a. Detailed sleep history taking:
      - Presleep routine
      - Sleep-wake pattern
      - Any sleep-related symptoms
      - Daytime symptoms
      - Identification of comorbid medical or psychiatric disorders
   b. Questionnaires and sleep logs and diaries:
      - Evaluation of daytime sleepiness: Epworth Sleepiness Scale
      - Psychological scales: Depression, anxiety, and stress scale
      - Dysfunctional beliefs and attitudes scale
      - Role of sleep diary: A sleep diary plays an important role in the diagnosis of insomnia. A sleep diary ideally is written prospectively; that is, it is written two times a day, and the notes are endorsed as early as possible, so the patient is advised to write about the daytime just before sleeping and about the nighttime immediately upon getting up.

         A retrospective recall of sleep and daytime habits leads to recall bias, and a generalization of the reporting might occur. Also, recall bias might cause underreporting or overreporting; hence it is important to make the sleep diary a prospective method rather than retrospective record.

A 2-week sleep diary can be studied for:

- Frequency of insomnia symptoms
- Type of symptom, i.e., the problem in sleep onset or maintenance of sleep, or a problem of waking up too early
- Duration of symptoms

For more details on a sleep diary, refer to Chapter 17, and for questionnaires and sleep interviews, refer to Chapters 15 and 16.

   c. Role of overnight polysomnography: In a case of insomnia alone, polysomnography is not necessary for diagnosis, but in patients where other disorders of sleep are suspected, polysomnography is indicated. PSG may be done if the patient remains refractory to insomnia therapy, gives a history of arousals associated with unexplained behavior, history of snoring, dryness in mouth, or witnessed apnea suggestive of obstructive sleep apnea, etc.

      Paradoxical insomnia is diagnosed using polysomnography.
   d. Role of actigraphy: Actigraphy is indicated only if there is suspicion of depression with insomnia. In cases where the circadian rhythm pattern is suspected to be affected along with insomnia, actigraphy may be preferable for 2 weeks.

2. **Treatment of insomnia**: The goals of therapy are to reduce the daytime consequences and improve sleep quality and quantity. Improvement in wake after sleep onset, sleep onset latency, sleep quality, sleep efficiency, total sleep time, or reduction in daytime distress and number of awakenings at night are considered specific goals of therapy in these patients. A better association formation of bed and sleep and better sleep-related psychological distress are also considered specific goals of therapy.

   There are two types of treatment approaches in these patients: pharmacological and nonpharmacological.
   a. Pharmacological approach to insomnia: Pharmacological treatment for insomnia is an important approach in a case of acute insomnia, initially as a support in chronic insomnia, acute painful conditions, or medical and psychiatric conditions requiring sleep treatment. A list of drugs depending on the results of the clinical trials can be found in the American Academy of Sleep Medicine (AASM) guidelines. These guidelines are based on the GRADE approach (Grades of Recommendation, Assessment, Development and Evaluation), where in the task force assessed the quality of evidence, balance of benefits and harms, patient's values, and preferences. For the assessment of quality of evidence, objective

data were used. Meta-analysis data were used for determining benefits and harms. The patient's values and preferences were formulated by using published data and clinical expertise.

Drugs recommended for sleep onset insomnia were found to reduce sleep latency in clinical trials. Recommended doses and side effects of each of them are given in the AASM guideline paper by Sateia et al. Sleep quality increased as compared to a placebo with eszopiclone, temazepam, triazolam, or zolpidem.

The task force listed drugs recommended as per AASM guidelines for sleep onset and sleep maintenance insomnia, along with drugs not recommended for insomnia, as shown here:

Dosage and duration should be carefully monitored by the physician. In case daytime sleepiness is affecting the patient's day-to-day activity, the clinician may conduct a review, and the drug may be changed. The pharmacological approach is of value in acute insomnia and in chronic insomnia while transitioning to CBTI. Sometimes long-term pharmacological support is required in chronic comorbid illnesses with insomnia.

b. Nonpharmacological approach for treatment of insomnia: As per the AASM guidelines, multicomponent cognitive behavioral therapy for chronic insomnia is strongly recommended. Depending on the clinical condition of the patient and solely at the discretion of the clinician only or due to the patient's preference, multicomponent

*Drugs Recommended for Sleep Onset Insomnia

Eszopiclone
Ramelteon
Temazepam
Triazolam
Zaleplon
Zolpidem

*Drugs Recommended for Sleep Maintenance Insomnia

Doxepin
Eszopiclone
Suvorexant
Zolpidem
Temazepam

*AASM Guidelines Sateia et al., 2017

*Drugs NOT Recommended for Sleep Onset or Sleep Maintenance Insomnia

Diphenhydramine
Melatonin
Tiagabine
Trazodone
L-tryptophan
Valerian

*AASM Guidelines Sateia et al., 2017

brief behavioral therapies, stimulus control or relaxation therapy, or sleep restriction as a single therapy may be advised.

The nonpharmacological approach to insomnia includes multicomponent cognitive behavioral therapy for insomnia (CBTI). It is strongly recommended even as a standalone therapy for chronic insomnia in adults. A typical multicomponent CBTI lasts approximately 4–8 sessions, during which the therapist identifies the maladaptive beliefs that are hampering patient's sleep. Various multicomponent are used like sleep restriction, sleep education, sleep hygiene, stimulus control, relaxation training, and cognitive restructuring in the various sessions. It is a goal-directed approach where the therapist builds a strategy to improve sleep using various components. The entire therapeutic intervention is monitored using a sleep diary or thought diary, and hence a supervision of the progress of the patient is maintained throughout the intervention.

The therapy usually is tolerated well. In some circumstances, however, fatigue, tiredness, daytime sleepiness, or attention problems might be precipitated because of sleep deprivation from sleep restriction. In such cases, sleep restriction should be best avoided. Sleep restriction is also contraindicated in patients with seizure disorder or bipolar disorder, which may precipitate due to effects of sleep deprivation. Suitability for CBTI should be judged by the therapist. Here are a few points to consider:

- The patient should be motivated to attend these sessions. It is important to check in the initial session whether the patient is willing to change the maladaptive behaviors that may be affecting sleep.
- In cases where specific problems may be identified, the therapy works better since specific treatment goals can be formulated and targeted during the therapy sessions.
- Patience is necessary by both the therapist and the patient as the progress of improvement is gradual and slow.
- In case the primary care physician feels that the patient just needs to talk, a counsellor may be suggested before CBTI.

- The physician also needs to understand the cost involved, feasibility in terms of distance of travel to reach a trained person, and time required while prescribing CBTI.
- In case the multicomponent therapy is not feasible due to the lack of a trained therapist, patients' availability, feasibility, etc., a brief therapy of 1–4 sessions can be taken, or stimulus control, relaxation therapy, or cognitive therapy as a single component may be taken with sleep education and sleep hygiene. Sleep hygiene alone, however, is not recommended in chronic insomnia patients.

Details of each component is laid out in Chapter 22 on nonpharmacological approach to sleep disorders.

In cases where insomnia remains a symptom and is clearly a disorder, multicomponent CBTI may be offered if the patient can afford it. Otherwise, brief multicomponent therapy or even single component therapies may be tried. Counselling may also help in identifying the problem and might help the individual to formulate a plan for future. Self-help books can also empower the patients to identify their own problems and find solutions such that the insomnia symptom can be resolved. One such book by the author is enclosed as further reading, which may be recommended by clinicians to enable their patients. Relaxation training using progressive muscular relaxation, meditation, or yoga nidra, may be tried under supervision.

Treatment of comorbidities, whether medical or psychiatric, or chronic painful conditions should be attended to. Other commonly seen coexisting sleep disorders like restless leg syndrome, obstructive sleep apnea, etc. should be ruled out.

REVIEW OF INSOMNIA PATIENTS

These patients should be reviewed weekly initially during the start of stabilization, then may be seen once every few weeks or monthly until they stabilize or resolve, after which the review can be done every 6 months, which is advocated since relapses are very common.

The broad outline of the clinical approach to a case of insomnia is shown in Figure 6.1.

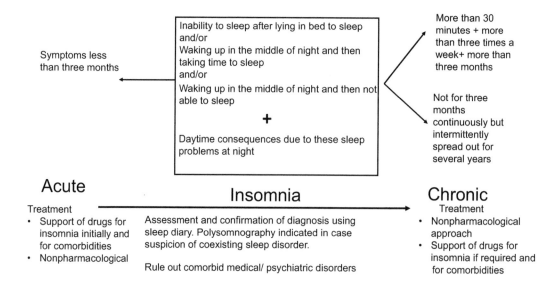

Figure 6.1 Broad outline of clinical approach to a case of insomnia.

SUGGESTED READING

1. Sateia MJ, Buysse DJ, Krystal AD, Neubauer DN, Heald JL. Clinical Practice Guideline for the Pharmacologic Treatment of Chronic Insomnia in Adults: an American Academy of Sleep Medicine Clinical Practice Guideline. J Clin Sleep Med. 2017;13(2):307–349. Published 2017 Feb 15. doi:10.5664/jcsm.6470.

2. American Academy of Sleep Medicine. *International Classification of Sleep Disorders*, 3rd ed. Darien, IL: American Academy of Sleep Medicine; 2014.

3. Sateia MJ. International classification of sleep disorders-third edition: highlights and modifications. *Chest*. 2014;146(5):1387–1394. http://doi.org/10.1378/chest.14-0970.

4. Edinger JD, Arnedt JT, Bertisch SM, et al. Behavioral and psychological treatments for chronic insomnia disorder in adults:

an American Academy of Sleep Medicine clinical practice guideline. *J Clin Sleep Med.* 2021;17(2):255–262. https://doi.org/10.5664/jcsm.8986.

5. Self-help book 'My Sleep Diary- Reflections within and Beyond' by Col Karuna Datta. www.amazon.in/My-Sleep-Diary-Reflections-Within-Beyond/dp/9389624630/ref=tmm_hrd_swatch_0?_encoding=UTF8&qid=&sr=

6. Schutte-Rodin S, Broch L, Buysse D, Dorsey C, Sateia M. Clinical guideline for the evaluation and management of chronic insomnia in adults. *J Clin Sleep Med.* 2008;4(5):487–504.

7. Datta K, Tripathi M, Mallick HN. *Yoga Nidra*: an innovative approach for management of chronic insomnia: a case report. Sleep Sci Pract 2017;1:7. https://doi.org/10.1186/s41606-017-0009-4.

7

Does the Patient Snore? Does the Patient Stop Breathing at Times during Sleep?

DEEPAK SHRIVASTAVA, AND RICHA SHRIVASTAVA

INTRODUCTION

Snoring is a common occurrence and may be an early sign of sleep disordered breathing during sleep. The spectrum of the sleep disordered breathing ranges from snoring to obstructive sleep apnea.

Snoring is the respiratory sound generated by soft tissue vibration in the upper airway during sleep. It is mostly generated during the inspiratory phase of breathing. Risk factors include male sex, being overweight or obese, increasing age, nasal obstruction, pregnancy, smoking, and use of substances that reduce muscle tone in the upper airway.

In patients with snoring without OSA and with BMI <30 kg/m2, the increased snoring index (snoring events/hour) is associated with increased all-cause mortality, according to the *Journal of Otolaryngology-Head & Neck Surgery* 2011.

THE DIFFERENT NAMES FOR SNORING

- Simple snoring
- Habitual snoring
- Isolated snoring
- Benign snoring
- Non-apneic snoring
- Socially disruptive snoring
- Non-sleepy snoring
- Continuous snoring
- Rhythmic snoring
- Non-dangerous snoring

Primary snoring is typically defined as snoring without any or with few episodes of apnea and hypopneas with an apnea hypopnea index (AHI)

DOI: 10.1201/9781003093381-9

of <5 events per hour of sleep or respiratory-event-related arousals as documented by sleep testing. In primary snoring, there is an absence of daytime sleepiness or insomnia

INCIDENCE AND PREVALENCE OF PRIMARY SNORING

- A wide variation is noted in the prevalence of snoring from 2 to 86% in different populations.
- One must realize that occasional snoring is nearly universal.
- According to the seminal Wisconsin sleep cohort study, the prevalence of snoring is 40% in men and 24% in women. However, different prevalences are documented in subsets of populations in other countries.

WHAT MAY PRESENT AS SNORING?

Snoring results from vibration caused by the partial or complete soft tissue obstruction of the upper airway by muscle tone relaxation, leading to oropharyngeal collapse due to alcohol, sedatives (such as diphenhydramine), narcotics, or other substances. Other nasal or sinus conditions (such as polyps, adenoidal hypertrophy, or nasopharyngeal masses) can contribute to snoring:

- Excess adipose tissue in the neck and throat is most noted in patients with obesity and overweight and can cause snoring episodes especially in supine body position.
- The incidence of tongue dropping into the airway due to the retrognathia (back set mandible), micrognathia (small mandible), macroglossia (large tongue or relatively large size of the tongue for the jaw).

RESTRICTION OF THE SOFT TISSUE STRUCTURES

- Large uvula
- Large or swollen tonsils
- Septum abnormalities, including perforation or other mucosal problems
- Soft tissue edema or inflammation secondary to smoking, allergies, infection, nasal or sinus conditions, including nasopharyngeal mass and growths, adenoidal hypertrophy or polyps

THE PATHOGENESIS OF SNORING

It is important to understand what causes the snoring sound. The sound is caused by the movement of air flowing through partially obstructed airways during sleep. The airflow is turbulent, and vibration of the pharyngeal soft tissue occurs, resulting in the sound production called snoring. In general, sound is produced during the inspiratory phase of the breathing but occasionally can persist into the expiratory phase.

RISK FACTORS FOR SNORING

- Male sex
- Overweight or obesity
- Increasing age
- Nasal obstruction
- Pregnancy
- Smoking
- Use of substances that reduce the muscle tone of the upper airway

EVALUATION FOR SNORING

A detailed history should include the history from the bed partner if possible and use of questionnaires to screen for possible obstructive sleep apnea.

Physical examination findings include a detailed assessment of the nose, oral cavity, and throat, neck circumference, and craniofacial features.

Assessment for obesity, craniofacial abnormalities, nasal septal deviation, Adenotonsillar hypertrophy, and nasal polyps may be obvious. Patients with nasal congestion may have nasal turbinate that appears boggy and edematous. The mucosal tissue is often erythematous or may have a pale bluish hue or pallor. The mucosa can also appear relatively normal.

Patients with acromegaly may manifest acral, articular, and soft tissue overgrowth, while patients with hypothyroidism may have delayed relaxation of deep tendon reflexes, bradycardia, coarse hair and skin, puffy facies, enlargement of the tongue, and hoarseness.

The diagnosis of primary snoring (PS) is based on ruling out obstructive sleep apnea (OSA); the upper airway resistance syndrome is considered part of OSA for diagnostic purposes by the American Academy of Sleep Medicine.

Additional testing may include a complete blood count to test for anemia, which may account for somnolence, and thyroid function testing to exclude hypothyroidism. Consider ECG to rule out underlying cardiovascular disease and testing for an underlying structural abnormality with testing for nasal airflow, such as with acoustic rhinometry, rhinomanometry, or rhino-resistometry.

Diagnostic testing for suspected craniofacial abnormalities or Adenotonsillar hypertrophy may include lateral cephalometric radiographs to provide information about the patency of the patient's upper airway.

COMPLICATIONS RELATED TO SNORING

Habitual snoring is associated with increased risk of stroke in an analysis of six studies with 126,427 participants (*International Journal of Cardiology* 2015 April 15; 185: 46).

Snoring has multiple potential consequences. Epidemiological studies show that snoring may be related to new onset hypertension, cardiovascular disease, and cerebrovascular disease. Snoring is also associated with carotid artery atherosclerosis. In an observational study, heavy snoring is noted to be associated with carotid artery atherosclerosis after adjustment for known confounders. There is a dose response relationship with prevalence of carotid atherosclerosis as 20% with mild, 32% with moderate, and 60% with heavy snoring. According to this study, there is a suggestion that snoring is associated with carotid atherosclerosis by itself. It is hypothesized that vibratory damage to the carotid artery walls from heavy snoring causes plaque formation and obstruction. This finding has been confirmed by other studies.

In another observational study of over 1400 subjects, polysomnography and blood pressure monitoring were done. Among individuals without obstructive sleep apnea, hypertension was equally likely among the heavy snorers and non-snorers. This study suggested that snoring alone is not associated with increased risk for high pressure. Multiple other studies also indicate that, in the absence of obstructive sleep apnea, snoring may not be independently associated with ischemic heart disease or all-cause mortality.

Snoring is associated with disrupted sleep of the bed partner and causes excessive daytime sleepiness and mental distress fraction according to multiple studies. A 2003 study published in *Chest* showed that OSA results in impaired quality of life for both the patient and her bed partner. Another 2008 study, published in the *Journal of Clinical Sleep Medicine*, showed that snoring intensity was independently related to sleepiness and apneic patients.

OFFICE MANAGEMENT OF SNORING

Lifestyle modification may include limiting alcohol consumption, smoke cessation, improving sleep hygiene, and avoiding medications that may cause snoring, for example, sleeping pills or hypnotics and sedating medications.

Smoking cessation is recommended for all patients. Elimination of alcohol consumption, especially during the several hours prior to bedtime, is recommended for patients who snore. In addition, improving sleep hygiene (such as maintaining a regular sleep-wake cycle, having a comfortable bed, and keeping the room dark and quiet) further reduces snoring.

If the probability of the obstructive sleep apnea is high based on the history and physical examination, the patient should be referred for evaluation by means of home sleep testing or in-lab sleep study for quantitative confirmation of the diagnosis.

Weight reduction and weight management are recommended for patients who are obese or overweight, as is weight loss for patients with obesity who snore since it may improve snoring. While most patients who lose weight see a reduction in snoring frequency, improvement is not universal and is unpredictable.

Myofunctional therapy includes oropharyngeal exercises to increase the muscle tone in the nasopharyngeal area. Oropharyngeal exercises for snoring may include tongue or palate exercises, singing, and/or instrument playing. Myofunctional therapy consists of combinations of oropharyngeal exercises and includes both isotonic and isometric exercises involving several muscles and areas of the mouth, pharynx, and upper respiratory tract in order to work on functions. Myofunctional therapy is associated with decreased snoring frequency, increased sleep quality, and reduced daytime sleepiness.

Pharmacologic therapy may include short-term use of nasal decongestant or steroids for chronic allergies. When snoring arises in association with acute sinusitis or rhinosinusitis, symptomatic measures to reduce nasal congestion before bedtime, such as saline nasal irrigation or intranasal decongestants, may help alleviate snoring. Topical decongestant use should be limited to 2–3 days because more prolonged use can induce rebound nasal congestion and rhinitis.

A trial of intranasal (topical) glucocorticoid therapy is recommended for patients with chronic nasal congestion and snoring.

Nasal dilators may be tried in patients with nasal airflow limitation. For patients who continue to snore despite conservative therapy and relief of any nasal congestion, a trial of using an external dilator is reasonable for most individuals who have snoring that is not associated with OSA and who continue to snore despite conservative interventions. Small studies have reported a decrease in either snoring frequency or intensity. Nonprescription nasal dilator strips may be beneficial and should be attempted in patients with nasal airflow restriction.

Note: Systemic medications and topical throat sprays are not recommended.

POSITIONAL THERAPY

Sleeping in the lateral position is a low-risk intervention that warrants a trial in most patients who snore. Body position therapy involves methods like using a pillow, backpack, a tennis ball sewn in the back of a shirt to facilitate sleeping in the non-supine position or to elevate the upper body.

Many commercial devices are now available in order to prevent patients sleeping on their backs. These include special pillows that are available with different modifications so that, turning on the back causes discomfort, leading to arousal. Positional alarms are available as well. Many simple devices can be made at home with a night shirt and tennis balls placed in the back pocket. The idea is to cause wakefulness when a person rolls over onto the back. Specialized pillows have been designed to keep the head in a position that keeps the airway open both when the person is lying on that side or on the back. Such devices decrease the intensity of snoring and reduce obstructive events in a few people.

NONOFFICE MANAGEMENT OF SNORING

Treatment of snoring by continuous positive airway pressure (CPAP) may be considered, but it is not routinely done due to poor acceptance and compliance problems, as well as higher cost associated with the use of CPAP therapy. In general, it is not covered by third-party payers or insurance for the snoring indication.

Specialist consultation, including a sleep specialist, dental sleep specialist, orthodontist, head and neck surgery, or ENT surgery, offer multiple interventions for the improvement of snoring on a case-by-case basis. At this point, the primary care provider may coordinate the care of the patient and acts as a patient advocate to facilitate the treatment plan.

In the event of surgical interventions for primary snoring, minimally invasive procedures should be favored over more invasive interventions. If nasal obstruction is the underlying cause of snoring, nasal surgery should be considered (such as septoplasty). Uvelopalatopharyngoplasty (UPPP) may be considered but is more invasive and has a higher rate of complications and morbidity. If the tongue base is the underlying cause of snoring, minimally invasive surgery at the tongue base (such as radiofrequency ablation) or on the tonsils may be considered. Invasive procedures outside the nose and soft palate are not recommended.

Drug-induced sleep endoscopy may be used for anatomical examination of the upper respiratory tract for primary snoring, the differentiation of primary snoring from OSA, or for help in selection of management options and may provide information about the site of airway obstruction.

The American Academy of Sleep Medicine/American Academy of Dental Sleep Medicine (AASM/AADSM) recommendations on oral appliance therapy for treatment of snoring suggest the use of oral appliances that protrude and stabilize the mandible rather than no therapy for adults requesting treatment of primary snoring without OSA. A follow-up with sleep testing by sleep physicians is suggested in adults who are prescribed oral appliances to improve or confirm treatment efficacy. Mandibular advancement devices are associated with reduced snoring.

IMPACT OF SNORING ON THE SLEEP OF THE BED PARTNER

- Annoyance and sleep disturbance
- Inability of the bed partner to sleep in the same room due to the noise of snoring
- Possible morning headaches and daytime sleepiness for the bed partner

SOME IMPORTANT FACTS TO CONSIDER

- The diagnosis of primary snoring is based on ruling out sleep disordered breathing (including obstructive sleep apnea) and upper airway resistance syndrome (respiratory-effort-related arousals [RERAs]).
- Diagnostic studies including in-lab nighttime polysomnography, home sleep testing, specialized endoscopies, radiologic studies including X-rays and cone beam CT, and testing for nasal airflow, e.g., acoustic rhinometry may further help establish the diagnosis in some cases.

SNORING CAN CAUSE COMPLICATIONS DURING PREGNANCY

- Chronic loud snoring may be associated with an increased rate of early delivery in pregnant patients without other comorbid conditions like high blood pressure or diabetes.
- Chronic snoring in third trimester pregnancies is known to be associated with increased risk of low birthweight and elective cesarean delivery.

PROGNOSIS IN PATIENTS WITH SNORING

Increased snoring may be associated with increased all-cause mortality in adults without obstructive sleep apnea and with body mass index <30 kg/m2. Snoring is associated with elevated markers of metabolic syndrome. Chronic mild inflammation and dysregulation are associated with the pathogenesis of obesity and other related metabolic disorders. It has been shown that C-reactive protein (CRP), fasting plasma glucose, lipid values, insulin, interleukin-6, adiponectin, and leptin were measured in patients who snored. Snoring was noted to be associated with heightened values of these inflammatory markers in this group of patients. The risk of metabolic syndrome was noted to be significantly high in regular snorers compared with nonsmokers.

SUGGESTED READING

1. Al Hussaini A, Berry S. An evidence-based approach to the management of snoring and adherence. *Clin Otolaryngol.* 2015;40(2):79–85.
2. Deary V. Simple snoring: not quite so simple after all? *Sleep Med Rev.* 2014; 18(6):453–462.
3. American Academy of Sleep Medicine. *International Classification of Sleep Disordered.* 3rd ed. Darien, IL: American Academy of Sleep Medicine; 2014.
4. Yaremchuk K. Why and when to treat snoring. *Otolaryngol Clin North Am.* 2020;53(3):351–365.

8

Does the Patient Have Excessive Daytime Sleepiness?

DEEPAK SHRIVASTAVA

APPROACH TO PATIENT WITH DAYTIME SLEEPINESS

Excessive daytime sleepiness is defined as difficulty staying awake during usual waking hours. The prevalence is estimated to be approximately 20% of the general population. Many conditions, including insufficient sleep, number of sleep-related breathing disorders, medications or substance use, psychiatric disorders, circadian rhythm disorders and excessive sleepiness due to central nervous system disorders, sleep-related movement disorders, metabolic disorders, and many medical conditions, may cause excessive daytime sleepiness (EDS).

Although what constitutes sleepiness would seem to be intuitively obvious, patients and providers may not always carefully distinguish true sleepiness (the propensity to fall asleep) from fatigue and/ or reduced alertness. Fatigue is characterized by a reduced ability to sustain effort and motivation. It is often perceived and referred to by patients as "tiredness" and is thus equated in their minds with sleepiness. This may lead to misinterpretation of the patient's complaint by their provider. Fatigue can be ameliorated by rest without necessarily sleeping, while sleepiness cannot. Alertness refers to the ability to sustain attention and includes a cognitive processing component. Although alertness is related to sleepiness in that sleepy persons may not be able to sustain attention, the two phenomena are not inextricably linked in a reciprocal manner. Persons with certain conditions—such as attention deficit hyperactivity disorder, depression, or psychosis—may

DOI: 10.1201/9781003093381-10

have a reduced ability to sustain attention but be fully awake and not sleepy.

In the office setting, determining whether an individual has abnormal sleepiness has two main purposes. First, it is important to determine whether sleepiness is compromising the patient's quality of life or putting him or her at risk for other health consequences. If so, determining the cause of the sleepiness and applying appropriate therapy are indicated and worthwhile.

Second, a provider has the responsibility to try to determine whether the level of sleepiness places the patient or society at risk for adverse consequences from inappropriate sleep episodes (e.g., an automobile crash caused by falling asleep while driving). The latter is a much more difficult task than the former, and neither standardized instruments for self-assessment nor objective tests of sleepiness have been shown to have high predictive value for risk.

The assessment of the risk for a drowsy-driving crash is especially important for patients with sleep disorders. Drowsy driving is common and often results in fatalities and serious injuries due to sleepiness. The high-risk group includes teenage drivers, patients with obstructive sleep apnea, shift workers, medical house staff, law enforcement officers, and commercial drivers. According to the National Sleep Foundation, approximately 60% of drivers confess admitting drowsy driving, and 40% in fact have fallen asleep while driving during the prior year. Of teenage drivers, 50–70% admitted to drowsy driving. Drowsy driving increases the relative risk of a motor vehicle crash by 2.5 times.

In order to evaluate the patient further, details regarding the patient's sleep history, past medical, psychiatric, and surgical and family history is required. In addition, a physical examination and sometimes appropriate laboratory testing are essential.

Patients may describe their sleepiness in many ways. In general, they may report a feeling of fatigue, lack of energy, feeling tired, lethargic, mood changes, and inability to concentrate. In addition, the assessment of their daytime energy levels is important to understand the impact of poor-quality sleep on their overall health.

The provider should ask questions about the effect of the sleepiness on the patient's daily activities, including the inability to stay alert at work, completing tasks at home, school performance, or drowsy driving, as well as history of any accidents.

The other sources of information, including caregivers and family members, may also provide significant information regarding snoring habits, choking or gasping for air during the sleep, and sleeping with an open mouth. Patients may further add waking up in the morning with a dry mouth, nasal congestion, and headaches, as well as excessive urination during the night (nocturia).

It is important to ask about sleeping patterns and sleepiness, including the time of sleep onset and offset, the time taken to fall asleep (sleep latency time), variability in sleep time during the weekend and holidays, and total sleep time in 24 hours including daytime naps, use of any sleep medications to fall asleep or the stimulant medication to stay awake during the daytime including caffeine consumption.

Special attention should be paid to the use of medications like benzodiazepine or opioids, seizure medications, antihistamines, neuroleptic medication, antidepressant and dopamine agonists. For many disorders, family history is important to obtain. This includes a history of narcolepsy, sleep apnea, restless leg syndrome, periodic leg movement disorders, major depression, or bipolar disorder

WHAT CAN BE DONE IN AN OFFICE SETTING TO EVALUATE THE PATIENT WITH EDS?

Patients generally use vague descriptive terms to report sleepiness, including fatigue, lack of energy, feeling tired, lethargy, moodiness, and difficulty concentrating. As a general approach to the further collection of information, questions about the effect of sleepiness on daily activities, including staying awake at work, completing chores at home, performance at school, or driving, including near-miss accidents, should be considered. How and what the patient, caregiver, and/or bed partner report about sleep-related symptoms suggestive of obstructive sleep apnea (OSA) are important, including episodes of loud snoring alternating with quiet episodes of pauses in breathing, dry mouth, nasal congestion, nocturnal enuresis, and morning headaches or other abnormal sleep conditions like restless legs syndrome or insomnia.

The primary physician needs to ask questions about the history of sleeping patterns and sleepiness, including time of sleep onset and offset, sleep latency, variability on the weekends, total sleep time (including naps), use of hypnotics to fall asleep or stimulants to stay awake, and daytime energy level. Medication history, with special attention to benzodiazepines, opioids, barbiturates, anticonvulsants, antihistamines, neuroleptics, dopamine agonists, and antidepressants, is always important as these medications have significant effects on different sleep stages and the sleep architecture.

A family history of narcolepsy, OSA, restless leg syndrome, periodic leg movement disorder, major depressive disorder, or bipolar disorder should be carefully solicited and documented. The severity of daytime sleepiness may be evaluated using a variety of instruments available for use in office settings.

Validated questionnaires like the Epworth sleepiness scale (ESS), Stanford Sleepiness Scale (SSS), and STOP-BANG Questionnaire are some examples of currently used screening tools. None of these subjective scales show strong correlations with objective measures of sleepiness. More importantly, increased scores on these self-rating scales are also not clearly associated with an increased risk of sleep-related adverse events, such as drowsy-driving crashes. Persons with sleep apnea who have had a motor vehicle crash in the previous 3 years and those who had not were found to have similar ESS scores.

WHAT ARE THE EXPECTED PHYSICAL EXAMINATION FINDINGS?

The physical examination may be unremarkable for any findings. However, for disorders like obstructive sleep apnea, the patient's body mass index (BMI) may suggest obesity; shallow rapid compensated breathing may suggest obesity hypoventilation syndrome and anhedonia; and flat affect or decreased mood may suggest major depressive disorder or bipolar disorder. Skin pallor may suggest underlying anemia. Dry coarse, cool yellowish skin, and coarse brittle hair and nails may suggest underlying hypothyroidism.

SPECIFIC FEATURES SUGGESTING OBSTRUCTIVE SLEEP APNEA

- Retrognathia (smaller back set mandible)
- Narrowing of the posterior pharynx
- Macroglossia, or large tongue relative to the size of the mouth
- Tonsillar hypertrophy or enlarged tonsils
- Elongated or enlarged uvula
- High arched or narrow hard palate
- Nasal abnormalities, including polyps, septal deviation, nasal valve abnormalities, or turbinate hypertrophy
- Overjet or protruding top incisors teeth up to more than 10 mm ahead of bottom incisors
- Large neck circumference (over 17 inches in men and over 16 inches in women), suggestive of obstructive sleep apnea
- Enlarged thyroid, suggestive of underlying hypothyroidism
- Nonpitting pretibial edema and brittle nails, suggestive of hypothyroidism
- Delayed tendon reflexes, suggestive of hypothyroidism

NONSPECIFIC SYMPTOMS ASSOCIATED WITH DAYTIME SLEEPINESS TO EXPLORE DURING THE PATIENT INTERVIEW

- Irritability
- Attention deficit and lack of concentration
- Reduced vigilance
- Easy distractibility
- Reduced motivation
- Low level of energy and generalized malaise
- Dysphoria
- Fatigue and tiredness
- Restlessness and agitation
- Lack of coordination

To assess the contributing causes of excessive daytime sleepiness, a review of the patient's current medications, including over-the-counter medications, herbal medications, and any substance use history, must be obtained.

In order to assess the circadian rhythm sleep-wake disorders, the following information may be obtained:

- Detailed information regarding the timing and rotation of shift work if the patient is a shift worker
- Patient's recent travel history and assessment for jet lag
- Patient experience of difficulty falling asleep at the usual and habitual sleep time and excessive morning sleep inertia or difficulty in waking up at the desired time may suggest delayed sleep phase disorder. (This information is crucial for college-age young adults.)
- History of sleeping too early and waking up too early in the morning and inability to get back to sleep may suggest advanced sleep phase syndrome. (This information is crucial for elderly individuals.)
- Intermittent symptoms of lack of sleep and excessive daytime sleepiness throughout 24 hours may suggest non-24-hour sleep-wake rhythm disorder. (And this disorder at sleep time and wake time is progressively delayed every day, and the disorder continues to cycle in a predictable pattern.)
- A recurrent pattern of irregular sleep and wake episodes throughout the 24-hours. Symptoms of insomnia at night and excessive daytime sleepiness during the day may suggest a regular sleep-wake rhythm disorder

DIAGNOSTIC TESTING INITIATED IN THE OFFICE AND CLINIC SETTINGS

Sleep- and wake-specific history and focused physical examination help to detect the presence of a sleep disorder and improve the pretest probability. Many symptoms are nonspecific and overlapping across a variety of sleep disorders. Based on a broad spectrum of differential diagnoses, a diagnostic plan can be formulated. The most appropriate diagnostic test is then ordered to establish the accurate diagnosis.

Sleep logs and actigraphy are common tools used for understanding sleep behavior and the patterns of individuals. Blood tests may be ordered for confirming the diagnosis of hyperthyroidism (TSH), anemia (hemoglobin), or restless leg syndrome (hemoglobin and serum ferritin levels). Urine toxicology may be obtained in order to assess the use of medications or illicit substances. If a seizure disorder is suspected of affecting the sleeping pattern, an electroencephalogram (EEG) may be ordered before referring the patient.

SLEEP LOG HELPS TO FACILITATE AND CONFIRM THE DIAGNOSIS

A sleep log can aid in facilitating and confirming the diagnosis of:

- Shift work sleep disorder.
- Delayed sleep phase syndrome.
- One sleep phase syndrome.
- Non-24 sleep-wake disorder.
- Irregular sleep-wake syndrome disorder.

ACTIGRAPHY MAY HELP FACILITATE AND CONFIRM THE DIAGNOSIS

Actigraphy is helpful in the following ways:

- Determination of the circadian pattern in patients with insomnia
- Determination of the circadian pattern in patients with hypersomnia
- Estimating the total sleep time in patients with suspected obstructive sleep apnea when polysomnography is not available
- Monitoring the sleep and circadian rhythm patterns in patients living in community or nursing homes where polysomnography is difficult to perform
- Assessing the sleep pattern of infants and children in the home, where polysomnography can be difficult to perform

Note: Actigraphy is not recommended for the evaluation of jet lag disorder (AASM guideline).

OBJECTIVE TESTS OF SLEEPINESS

Multiple Sleep Latency Test

The multiple sleep latency test (MSLT) was developed to quantify sleepiness, i.e., the propensity to fall asleep, in young healthy subjects participating in sleep restriction studies. The procedure recommended by the American Academy of Sleep Medicine (AASM) is that the subject or patient lies in bed in a darkened room with the instruction, "Try to fall asleep." Five nap opportunities are performed at 2-hour intervals starting 1.5 to 3 hours, after the termination of an overnight sleep study. Each nap period is terminated after 20 minutes if no sleep occurs or 15 minutes after the onset of any stage of sleep documented on EEG. Sleep onset latency is the time from lights out to the first epoch of sleep. An average of the sleep latencies for the nap periods is calculated using 20 minutes for any period in which no sleep occurred; this average is reported as the mean sleep latency (MSL) for the MSLT. The MSL on the MSLT is believed to measure the physiologic propensity for sleep in the absence of alerting factors. The manifest sleep tendency is likely determined by an interaction of many external factors (such as light, noise, and temperature), the individual's activity level, and internal factors affecting the level of activation of the arousal system (such as perceived stress, anxiety, and motivation).

The MSLT measures sleep propensity only on a given day under carefully controlled environmental conditions, so it may not accurately reflect an individual's sleep propensity under different circumstances or an overall average sleep propensity. This is given as a possible reason why the MSL on the MSLT does not correlate closely with an individual's score on the ESS. Also, individuals may have "high sleepability" when trying to fall asleep but also an ability to maintain wakefulness when attempting to do so (e.g., on the maintenance of wakefulness test [MWT]). The MSL on MSLT may be sensitive not only to the state (i.e., current) level of CNS arousal but also the trait (i.e., chronic) level.

Maintenance of Wakefulness Test (MWT)

The MWT consists of four nap periods at 2-hour intervals with the first trial beginning 1.5–3 hours after the subject/patient's usual wake-up time. The subject/patient is seated in a bed in a darkened room and instructed to "remain awake as long as possible." The subject/patient is not allowed to perform any specific maneuvers to try to stay awake (e.g., singing, pinching oneself, and so forth). Nap periods are ended after 20–40 minutes (the AASM

recommends using 40 minutes) if no sleep occurs or after unequivocal sleep (defined as 3 consecutive epochs of stage 1 sleep or 1 epoch of any other stage of sleep on EEG) occurs.

1. INSUFFICIENT SLEEP SYNDROME AND CENTRAL DISORDERS OF HYPERSOMNOLENCE

Sleep characteristics associated with insufficient sleep syndrome include unimpaired or above average ability to initiate and maintain sleep. In general, EDS in such conditions is a result of the following disorders.

Chronic sleep deprivation due to reduced time in bed is common in modern lifestyle. The patient is often unaware of insufficient sleep. Sleep deprivation due to insufficient time in bed may cause symptoms of sleep paralysis and hypnagogic hallucinations.

The central disorders of excessive sleepiness include multiple conditions with overlapping symptoms. In the case of narcolepsy, there are daily periods of an irrepressible need to sleep or daytime lapses into sleep. There are short, refreshing daytime naps and rapid eye movement sleep dissociation, including cataplexy (type 1 only), sleep paralysis, and hypnagogic or hypnopompic hallucinations. In addition, these patients have nocturnal sleep disruption with frequent awakenings. In idiopathic hypersomnia, patients report long, unwanted, unrefreshing naps (≥1 hour), difficulty waking up from naps, and sleep inertia (sleep drunkenness). These patients rarely have sleep paralysis and hallucinations. In another condition of central hypersomnia called Kleine–Levin syndrome, there are recurrent episodes with severe sleepiness lasting 2 days to several weeks, and they tend to recur once annually and about once every 18 months. Patients have normal sleep and behavior between episodes. Common presentations during symptomatic periods include the feeling of derealization or déjà-vu, hyperphagia, hypersexuality, and, less frequently, anorexia. During the active episode, patients have long 24-hour sleep times, personality changes, poor social interaction, confusion, and apathy.

2. CIRCADIAN RHYTHM SLEEP-WAKE DISORDERS

Circadian rhythm sleep disorders can lead to excessive daytime sleepiness. Common circadian rhythm disorders include characteristics associated with shift work disorder such as insomnia and unsatisfactory sleep quality; jet lag causing insomnia and disturbed sleep; delayed sleep-wake phase disorder, with difficulty falling asleep at the desired time; and excessive sleep inertia in the morning/difficulty waking at the desired time; and uncommon advanced sleep-wake phase disorder manifesting in early morning or maintenance insomnia (difficulty staying asleep or waking too early with inability to get back to sleep) and excessive evening sleepiness.

Other circadian rhythm sleep disorders include non-24-hour sleep-wake rhythm disorder, presenting with intermittent symptoms of insomnia or excessive daytime sleepiness, irregular sleep-wake rhythm disorder, a recurrent pattern of irregular sleep and wake episodes throughout a 24-hour period, and symptoms of insomnia at night with excessive sleepiness (napping) during the day.

Many psychiatric disorders, including seasonal affective disorder, tend to occur during fall and winter. The associated symptoms include depression and feelings of sadness, lack of energy, decreased level of activity, and craving for carbohydrate-rich food. During these episodes, patients gain weight and develop recurrent thoughts of death. The major depressive disorder demonstrates multiple unexplained symptoms, dampened affect, and changes in interpersonal relationships and dysfunctions. These patients also have memory problems and difficulty concentrating and making decisions. Similar and overlapping symptoms are found in bipolar disorders as well as somatic symptom disorders. In such cases, the intensity of symptoms appears out of proportion to the healthy appearance of the patient.

Multiple neurologic disorders include chronic fatigue syndrome, Alzheimer's dementia, Parkinson's disease, seizures, traumatic brain injury, and multiple sclerosis.

Many sleep-related movement disorders include restless leg syndrome, and the movement disorder can also cause excessive daytime sleepiness.

WHEN TO REFER A PATIENT WITH EDS TO A SLEEP SPECIALIST

Approximately 80 different sleep disorders affect the general population. It is estimated that 40 million Americans have one or another sleep disorder. Regardless of the disorder, the poor quality of sleep or insufficient sleep leads to significant health problems, including high blood pressure, diabetes, obesity, cardiovascular disease, and mental health problems, such as stress, problems with attention, concentration, and memory, and an irresistible urge to sleep at inappropriate times. While some of these disorders can be addressed by the primary care provider, the management of such disorders is complex and/or require specialized testing including a nocturnal sleep study, also known as polysomnography, a multiple sleep latency test, or maintenance of a fullness test. Many patients require continued follow-up with a sleep specialist for ongoing management of their disorders. Sleep specialists are in a better position to make further referrals for surgical intervention or continued medical management.

In the case of the unavailability of sleep specialists, consider referring the patient to a pulmonary specialist, neurology specialist, or psychiatric specialist with experience and interest in the practice of sleep medicine.

For the confirmation of the diagnosis and management recommendation, consider:

- A polysomnography test, also known as an overnight sleep study.
- Evaluation and management of alveolar hypoventilation syndrome.
- Evaluation and management of movement disorders of sleep.
- Further evaluation and management of difficult parasomnias and seizure disorders.
- Evaluation with EEG and other specialized techniques with simultaneous video recording of the patient's nocturnal behavior and movements.
- Evaluation and management of symptoms consistent with narcolepsy that include excessive daytime sleepiness, cataplexy (sudden loss of muscle tone), sleep paralysis, and sleep onset or sleep offset hallucinations.

CONCLUSION

Once the cause of excessive daytime sleepiness is determined, then a cause-specific management plan is recommended. The overall management of insufficient sleep includes longer hours of sleep based on the best total sleep time. The total sleep time is variable for different age groups. It must be realized that individual variability in sleep need may be influenced by genetic, behavioral, medical, and environmental factors. Therefore, patients should be counseled regarding behavioral strategies, the safety risks, and the medication risk associated with sleep disorders.

9

Does the Patient Have Abnormal Movements at Night?

DEEPAK SHRIVASTAVA

SLEEP-RELATED MOVEMENT DISORDERS

- RLS (restless legs syndrome)
- PLMD (periodic limb movement disorder)
- Leg cramps
- Bruxism
- Rhythmic movement disorders

RESTLESS LEG SYNDROME (RLS)

RLS is a disorder characterized by an irresistible urge to move the legs that worsens at rest and predominantly occurs in the evening or at night. The discomfort improves with movement. Patients present with unpleasant leg sensations at bedtime that disturb and delay sleep onset and disrupt sleep. These unpleasant sensations may be described as "creepy crawling," "burning," or "itching." The most common complaint in general is a sense of restlessness and a desire to move. The disrupted sleep may lead to a complaint of insomnia or daytime sleepiness. The discomfort most commonly involves the lower extremities but has been described in the upper extremities and even the torso. RLS has a circadian predominance. Symptoms tend to intensify in the evening or little later in the night. Movement like stretching or walking relieves the symptoms.

DOI: 10.1201/9781003093381-11

The prevalence is 5–10% of the general population and is more common in women with advancing age. About 21–57% of patients also describe upper extremity arm sensations. It can occur in multiple medical conditions including chronic renal failure, pregnancy, and iron deficiency (*International Classification of Sleep Disorders*, 3rd edition).

RLS remains underdiagnosed, but the prevalence of RLS appears to be in the 10–15% range for all adults and increases with age. The requirement that the leg discomfort occurs at least twice a week and is of moderate to severe intensity results in a prevalence of 2–4%. Women are about twice as likely as men to report RLS. Women who have had three or more children are at increased risk for RLS compared with their nulliparous sisters. A familial tendency is recognized for the development of both RLS and periodic limb movements.

Multiple medications, including tricyclic antidepressants, lithium, dopamine agonist, antipsychotics, and antiemetics, as well as selective serotonin reuptake inhibitors (SSRI), increase symptoms of RLS and periodic limb movements. Many lifestyle changes, including obesity and active lifestyle, nicotine use, caffeine, are associated with the symptoms of RLS.

The evaluation includes testing for iron deficiency, folate deficiency, vitamin B12 deficiency, diabetes, kidney disease, and thyroid dysfunction. The diagnosis of RLS is made by means of a history without the need for a formal sleep study.

Specifically Included Diagnostic Criteria for RLS

- The unpleasant sensation starts in the legs during periods of rest or inactivity.
- The sensation is relieved by movement, such as walking or stretching.
- It occurs exclusively during the night or evening.
- There is an urge to move the legs often, accompanied by discomfort and an unpleasant sensation in the legs.

Primary Care Management of RLS

Restless leg syndrome (RLS) can be treated with both nonpharmacologic and pharmacologic approaches. In fact, both approaches are combined for greater successful results. Pharmacologic treatment is based on medications like ropinirole and pramipexole, both dopamine receptor agonists that are FDA approved as a first-line treatment for RLS. Alternate medications include gabapentin and pregabalin. Other medications that have been used is rotigotine and levodopa. Opiates play a significant role in the management of refractory RLS. Both oxycodone and naloxone have been used in this situation.

Nonpharmacologic measures are generally supportive and include avoiding smoking and alcohol consumption, education regarding lifestyle, moderate exercise, and review of the medications that may be involved in worsening the RLS symptoms. An important intervention is to measure serum ferritin levels, and if anemia is present, iron supplementation should be instituted.

Refractory restless leg syndrome symptoms that are not responsive to the pharmacologic agents just mentioned may be treated with opioid medications with extended-release oxycodone/naloxone. However, the risks associated with long-term opioid use should be considered before subjecting the patient to therapy.

Primary Care Management of PLMD

Periodic limb movements are the rhythmic movements of the lower extremity with the dorsiflexion of the ankle, extension of the rectal and flexion of the knee and hip. They tend to occur at the first part of the night. Periodic limb movements increase in frequency with increasing age. Typical, periodic limb movements last approximately 2–4 seconds and occur every 20–40 seconds.

Other Names for PLMD

- Periodic movement disorders of sleep
- Sleep myoclonus syndrome
- Nocturnal myoclonus syndrome (*International Classification of Sleep Disorders*, 3rd edition)

Diagnostic Criteria for PLMD

To diagnose periodic limb movements, specific criteria are available. Include a series of 4 or more movements, each lasting 0.5–5 seconds at a frequency interval of 4–90 seconds. More than 15 events per hour of sleep are considered high and are diagnostic of periodic limb movement disorder in the correct clinical setting.

- Demonstration of periodic limb movements (PLMs) during sleep by polysomnography, also known as overnight in lab sleep study.
- Frequency of >5 PLMs/hour of sleep in children and >15 PLMs/hour in adults.
- Periodic leg movements (PMLs) can result in clinically significant sleep disturbance or impaired mental, physical, social, occupational, educational, behavioral, and other important areas of functioning.

Primary Care Management of PLMD

Periodic limb movement during sleep can occur with the presence of other sleep disorders. Most patients with RLS have associated PLMs. In addition, other disorders, like upper airway resistance syndrome, sleep disordered breathing narcolepsy, and RBD, are associated with increased PLMs. When these movements disrupt sleep and cause sleep fragmentation, resulting in daytime sleepiness or nighttime insomnia, the condition is referred to as periodic limb movement disorder (PLMD). Once identified, this disorder can be quite disabling and should be treated immediately with both nonpharmacologic, and pharmacologic therapy as previously outlined. Refractory and difficult cases should be referred to a sleep specialist. If the sleep specialist is not available, the patient should be referred to neurology.

SLEEP-RELATED LEG CRAMPS

In general population, these are very common, sudden, involuntary, and painful muscle contractions that usually involve calf muscles and small muscles of the foot that occur while resting, usually while sleeping. The symptoms are common, and the frequency of cramps increases with age

Other Names for Sleep-related Leg Cramps

- Leg cramps
- Charley horse
- Nocturnal leg cramps
- Nocturnal muscle cramps
- Nighttime leg cramps

Common Medical Conditions and Medications Associated with Leg Cramps

- Diabetes mellitus
- Peripheral vascular disease
- Hypokalemia
- Hypocalcemia
- Prolonged standing
- Oral contraceptives
- IV iron sucrose (*International Classification of Sleep Disorders*, 3rd edition)

Diagnostic Criteria

- Painful sensation in the leg or foot that is associated with sudden, involuntary muscle hardness or tightness, indicating a strong muscle contraction
- Painful muscle contraction while in bed asleep or awake
- Pain relieved by releasing the muscle contraction by forceful stretching

Primary Care Management

No treatments have been known to be reliably effective and safe. Address the potential causes including the underlying medical condition or the medications that may be responsible for causing nocturnal leg cramps. Consider a trial of stretching, mild exercise, and massage with forced dorsiflexion of the foot with the knee extended while massaging the calf muscle. There is no evidence to support pharmacologic treatment for nocturnal leg cramps in nonpregnant patients. Some studies show the beneficial use of vitamin B complex or diltiazem. For pregnant women with nocturnal leg cramps, a trial of oral magnesium for more than 3 weeks, vitamin B, and calcium may reduce leg cramps.

Note: The FDA recommends against the use of quinine for leg cramps due to its serious side effects.

SLEEP-RELATED BRUXISM

Sleep-related bruxism is defined by repetitive jaw muscle activity during sleep, manifested by the clenching or grinding of teeth and by the bracing or thrusting of the mandible. The prevalence of sleep-related bruxism is highest during childhood and is approximately 14–17% in the general population. It usually presents with tooth damage, pain, or disturbing sounds of teeth grinding.

Other Names for Bruxism

- Nocturnal bruxism
- Nocturnal teeth grinding
- Tooth clenching (*International Classification of Sleep Disorders*, 3rd edition)

Diagnostic Criteria

- Presence of regular or frequent tooth grinding sounds during sleep
- One or more of the following clinical signs and symptoms:
  - Abnormal tooth wear consistent with tooth grinding during sleep
  - Transient morning jaw muscle pain or fatigue, temporal headache, and jaw locking upon waking up

Primary Care Management

Over-the-counter mouth guards may protect tooth damage. If anxiety and stress are the cause of bruxism, then a referral to a counsellor may be made. If bruxism is severe and causes daytime symptoms including gum pain, tooth damage, and daytime fatigue due to poor nighttime sleep, then the patient should be referred to a dental sleep specialist or sleep specialist.

SLEEP-RELATED RHYTHMIC MOVEMENT DISORDER

Sleep-related rhythmic movement disorder is characterized by repetitive, stereotyped, and rhythmic motor behaviors that occur mainly during drowsiness or sleep and involve large muscle groups. They are most common in infants and children. Sleep-related rhythmic movements are without significant consequences except when there is risk of injury due to the intensity of the movement.

The onset typically occurs within the first 2 years of life and may affect up to 20% of healthy children. Persistence into adulthood is rare and may be associated with significant psychopathological disorders, such as autism. The male-to-female ratio is approximately 3:1. Rare complications resulting from these movements, when very severe, may include skull callus, retinal petechiae, and subdural hemorrhage.

Rhythmic movement episodes (movement artifacts) during any stage of sleep or wakefulness and the absence of seizure activity in association with the disorder are shown on polysomnography. Video monitoring may reveal stereotyped movements comprising rhythmic oscillation of the head and limbs. The rhythm frequency is between 0.5 and 2 Hz in long clusters with rhythmic "chanting" and other vocalization. Head banging is more likely to be present during REM sleep, while body rocking is more likely to be present during light sleep (stages 1 and 2). In the diagnostic workup of these episodes, one should assess for any underlying neurologic or psychiatric disorder that may cause the symptoms (i.e., nocturnal epilepsy). The differential diagnosis includes bruxism, thumb sucking, PLMS, and infantile spasms. When adults manifest RMD, consideration should be given to neurologic or psychiatric causes.

Other Names for Sleep-related Rhythmic Movement Disorder

- Body rocking
- Head banging
- Head rolling
- Body rolling (*International Classification of Sleep Disorders*, 3rd edition)

Diagnostic Criteria

- Repetitive, stereotyped, and rhythmic motor behaviors involving large muscle groups
- Sleep-related movements occurring near nap or bedtime or when individual appears drowsy or asleep
- Movement resulting in >1 of the following:
  - Sleep interference
  - Significant impairment in daytime function
  - Self-inflicted injury or potential self-inflicted injury if left untreated
- No better explanation by another movement disorder or epilepsy

Primary Care Management

Treatment is often not necessary. Parents may consider the use of bed padding and a protective helmet if the episodes lead to excessive noise or bodily injury. Behavioral modification may be used, as well as, if the episodes are severe, short-acting benzodiazepines or TCAs. Reassurance to the parents is the single best intervention. In more complicated cases involving parents with high anxiety levels, a referral to a sleep specialist should be considered.

PROPRIOSPINAL MYOCLONUS AT SLEEP ONSET

Propriospinal myoclonus at sleep onset is a disorder characterized by sudden, usually spontaneous myoclonic jerks occurring while falling asleep and rarely during intrasleep wakefulness and waking up in the morning. The prevalence of this disorder is noted to be 16–20% in the general population and is associated with a structural spinal cord pathology. They are more common in men and have not been reported in children (*International Classification of Sleep Disorders, 3rd edition*).

Diagnostic Criteria

- Presence of sudden jerks, especially of abdomen, trunk, and neck
- Evidence of jerks during relaxed wakefulness and drowsiness, when patient is falling asleep
- Disappearance of jerks upon mental activation and during stable sleep
- Jerks resulting in difficulty falling asleep

PARASOMNIAS PRESENTING AS SLEEP MOVEMENT DISORDERS

Confusional arousals usually take place following arousals from sleep, most typically deep sleep in the first part of the night. Episodes may last several minutes, often with absence of recollection of mental activity. They represent an admixture of wakefulness into non-REM sleep. Patients partially awaken and exhibit marked confusion, slow mentation, disorientation, perceptual impairment, and errors of logic. The memory for the event is often absent.

Sleepwalking is a series of complex behaviors that are initiated during slow wave sleep (SWS) that result in walking during sleep. Communication with the patient is often difficult. The behaviors may range widely, be of a repetitive nature, and have a symbolic meaning. The main concern with this parasomnia is the risk of injury. Patients may engage in activities that may produce cuts and bruises from bumping into objects or falling. Sleepwalking often lasts 1–5 minutes, but, rarely, episodes may last more than an hour if behavioral spells are complex. Hybrid attacks may occur, during which time sleep terrors precede and evolve into the sleepwalking.

Sleep terrors are a syndrome that consist of a sudden arousal from deep sleep manifested by a piercing scream or cry and accompanied by significant autonomic and behavioral manifestations of intense fear. It is the most dramatic of arousal disorders. It is often an extreme autonomic arousal. When a spell occurs, one may see elevated sympathetic activity manifested by tachycardia; tachypnea; reduced skin resistance, reflecting diaphoresis; flushing of the skin; mydriasis; and decreased and increased muscle tone. Sleep terrors often may be accompanied by incoherent vocalizations or micturition. There may be variable motor activity such as extreme agitation or escape behavior. These are states of cerebral hyperresponsiveness. The spells may be dangerous, as patients may hurt themselves during the escape behavior.

SLEEP-RELATED MOVEMENT DISORDER DUE TO MEDICAL DISORDER

The diagnosis for sleep-related movement disorder due to medical disorder is used for sleep-related movement disorders due to underlying conditions and not meeting criteria for any other movement disorder. The diagnosis of sleep-related movement disorder due to a medication or substance is used for a sleep-related movement disorder due to medication or a substance and not meeting the criteria for any other movement disorder. Examples of such disorders may be posttraumatic stress disorder (PTSD) and nightmares.

Disturbances in the normal sleep pattern and circadian rhythm are the major features of movement disorders, with the resultant exacerbation of motor or nonmotor symptoms as well as those of cardiac life. To provide the best care to patients with sleep disturbances, an understanding of these disorders is extremely important. In addition to abnormal sleep circadian rhythm patterns, side effects from the medications can also aggravate or cause many of these disorders. To better manage sleep-related movement disorders, it is imperative to understand the nature and the temporal pattern of the sleep across the spectrum of the many movement disorders.

SUGGESTED READING

1. American Academy of Sleep Medicine. *International Classification of Sleep Disorders*, 3rd ed. Darien, IL: American Academy of Sleep Medicine; 2014.
2. Bailey GA, Hubbard EK, Fasano A, et al. Sleep disturbance in movement disorders: insights, treatments and challenges. *J Neurol Neurosurg Psychiatry*. 2021;92:723–736.
3. Rana, AQ, Khan, F, Mosabbir, A, Ondo, W. Differentiating nocturnal leg cramps and restless legs syndrome. *Expert Rev Neurother*. 2014;14(7):813–818.
4. Silber MH. Sleep-related movement disorders. *Continuum (Minneap Minn)*. 2013;19(1 Sleep Disorders):170–184.

10

Does the Patient Have Pain, Headaches, High Blood Pressure, Diabetes, Stroke, Ventilation or Cardiac Disorders, or Other Problems?

KARUNA DATTA

INTRODUCTION

A patient reporting sleep complaints might have any kind of comorbid problem. It is very likely that the patient comes seeking for treatment of one or a combination of complaints or diseases like chronic pain, cardiac complaints of palpitations, exertional dyspnea, orthopnea, chest pain, breathing difficulty, tachypnea, hemiplegia, slurring of speech, with a history of hypertension, diabetes, etc. and, during history taking, gives a history of sleep complaints. In either of the conditions, if the sleep problem has a history of long duration, it becomes rather difficult to pinpoint which of the complaints came earlier. In other words, what was the cause or what was the effect is difficult to ascertain.

The aim of this chapter is to make the primary care physician conversant with the sleep problems or disorders commonly found in other disorders and the comorbidities that may coexist with sleep disorders. These common complaints need a thorough checkup and need a separate management plan.

PAIN COMPLAINTS AND SLEEP

One of the most troublesome complaints for which patient seeks treatment is pain. The International Association for the Study of Pain defines pain "as an unpleasant sensory and emotional experience associated with actual or potential tissue damage." Pain can be acute or chronic, somatic, or visceral and leads to sleep disruption. The exact mechanism by which pain causes sleep problems is not very clear, but it is proposed that pain is a protective mechanism and the activation of its pathway causes arousal. Sleep complaints caused by acute pain are found to be reversible, i.e., as the acute pain resolves, sleep also becomes better, and the problem resolves. Chronic pain, however, causes sleep problems that become a distinct entity and require specific management. Chronic pain effects last long and are associated with anxiety, fatigue, daytime sleepiness, impaired daytime performance, feeling of unwell, depression, and other somatic and cognitive dysfunction complaints.

DOI: 10.1201/9781003093381-12

Chronic pain is found to be commonly associated with sleep disorders like insomnia, periodic limb movement disorder (PLMD), and sleep disordered breathing (SDB). There may be the delayed onset of sleep or sleep may be disrupted throughout the night with frequent arousals and awakenings. Shifts between the sleep stages are increased, and studies find that slow wave sleep duration may also be reduced.

There is a correlation of sleep duration with the sensitivity of pain where sleep deprivation studies have proposed certain mechanisms. The studies propound that the sensitivity of pain may be affected due to a probable dysfunctional perception as is found in fibromyalgia. The various mechanisms for this increased sensitivity to pain are proposed by altered nociceptor sensitivity, altered endogenous pain inhibition mechanisms, and descending cortical mechanisms. Some patients also complain of allodynia, i.e., even non-nociceptive stimuli are perceived as painful stimuli.

Thus a patient suffering from chronic pain often reports sleep complaints. In outpatients, taking care of sleep problems is important not only because they need to be managed separately but also because, unless sleep improves, these patients do not feel well.

Management of Sleep

- The patient should be asked to maintain a sleep diary. A two-week sleep diary can provide adequate information about the waxing and waning of sleep complaints, if any, and give insight into the patient's sleep hygiene, as some factors might deteriorate patient's sleep like alcohol, meal timings, time of exercise, and its duration. The patient may also report nightmares or might remember a sensation of pain-related dreams. For details on how to instruct the patient regarding the filling out of sleep diary, see Chapter 17.
- If the patient has a problem initiating sleep or maintaining sleep, factors that may be responsible for increased arousal need to be identified. Any predisposing, perpetuating, and precipitating factors that affect the patient need to be identified. External factors like the room, comfort of the bed, or ambient noise and lighting must be made conducive for sleep. Nonpharmacological strategies work best for these patients in the long run. Initial or intermittent pharmacological support may be considered. AASM guidelines recommend eszopiclone, ramelteon, temazepam, triazolam, zaleplon, and zolpidem for sleep onset insomnia. For sleep maintenance insomnia, drugs recommended by AASM are doxepin, eszopiclone, suvorexant, zolpidem, and temazepam. A note must be made of the drugs not recommended by AASM: diphenhydramine, melatonin, tiagabine, trazodone, L-tryptophan, and valerian.
- Care must be taken to instruct and warn the individual in case a person has effects of drowsiness the next day. Geriatric patients tend to fall, and hence careful choice of drug with short action and the least residual drowsiness should be chosen. For better compliance, it is important to emphasize to the patient the role of the nonpharmacological approach in managing sleep problems.
- Also, management for pain is required as the cause and improvement in pain contribute to the patient's overall well-being.
- For more details on the nonpharmacological approach, please refer to Chapter 22.
- The assessment of pain may be done throughout the course of management using visual analog scales and validated questionnaires for pain and sleep. Since the effect of nonpharmacological management is gradual and takes time, it is important to record the scores for better management and follow-up of patient.

CARDIAC COMPLAINTS AND SLEEP

Apart from these conditions that cause pain and thus disrupt sleep, many other disorders may affect sleep due to physiological alterations. The cardiovascular and autonomic systems interact during sleep. During the initial stages of sleep, there is parasympathetic predominance, and baroreceptor gain is high leading to stability of blood pressure. Usually, a dip in blood pressure of approximately 10% during NREM sleep is found. In fact, cases that show less than a 10% dip in night blood pressure are called non-Dippers and have an increased risk for cardiovascular mortality, arrythmias, myocardial infarction, etc. Muscle sympathetic nerve activity is almost halved in slow wave sleep as compared to awake. At the time of transit between NREM to

REM, bursts of vagal nerve activity are seen that might cause a sudden reduction of heart rate and thus asystole are commonly seen. With the onset of REM, heart rate and blood pressure begin to rise and often fluctuate during REM. Patients with coronary artery disease, postmyocardial infarction, and diabetes are found to have a higher sympathetic drive during sleep as compared to normal volunteers. This increase further increases during REM sleep.

The effect of sympathetic drive on the heart causes an increase in heart rate (chronotropic), increased excitability (bathmotropic), increased contractility (ionotropic), increased conduction velocity of the signal (dromotropic), and increased rate of relaxation (lusitropic) of cardiac muscle. An increased sympathetic drive increases the myocardial oxygen demand required to be met by coronary circulation. The coronary blood flow to left side of the heart is predominantly during diastole, the duration of which is directly determined by the heart rate. As the heart rate increases, the duration of one beat is reduced, thereby further shortening the duration of diastole, and thus the heart rate becomes a major limiting factor. If the heart is diseased, this increase in oxygen demand cannot be met, leading to ischemia. This demand:supply ratio may be affected due to a greater than normal sympathetic drive, endothelial damage of the arteries, and an already diseased heart. High sympathetic drive is seen in post-myocardial infarction cases, and therefore vulnerability to arrhythmias and ischemic events is high in these cases, and they lead to sleep disturbances. Cardiac arrhythmias are seen during both REM and NREM due to alterations in the sympathetic and parasympathetic drive as discussed.

During NREM, there is a slight reduction in the sympathetic drive as compared to awake and REM sleep. The reduction in sympathetic drive causes reduction in volume and velocity of blood flow. During sleep, the prothrombotic milieu prevails, and in the background of vascular endothelial damage, NREM sleep serves as the right time when reduced blood velocity causes stagnation of blood and a predilection to the development of thrombi or dislodged emboli exists. Non-demand myocardial infarction during NREM is seen in patients with severe coronary disease, diabetes, and other causes of significant endothelial dysfunction.

COMMON ASSOCIATION OF CARDIOVASCULAR, NEUROLOGICAL, ENDOCRINAL DISORDERS WITH SLEEP

Cardiovascular disorders are commonly associated with sleep apnea. Obstructive sleep apnea is associated with endothelial dysfunction, hypertension, heart failure, arrhythmias, carotid artery stenosis, coronary artery disease, stroke and complications associated with change in autonomic function, and hormonal and metabolic function leading to increased morbidity and mortality.

In REM sleep, ventricular premature beats are commonly seen, and sinus bradycardia and even asystole might be seen during NREM sleep. Asystole is found in patients with cardiac disease on Class III antiarrhythmics. It is advisable to ascertain the absence of these pauses during sleep before starting this class of drugs.

Cases on lipophilic beta blockers, e.g., pindolol, metoprolol, and propranolol might complain of increased awakenings and increased wake after sleep onset due to the direct effect of the drug. A history of bizarre dreams and nightmares is also reported, along with daytime dysfunction like sleepiness and fatigue. Centrally acting alpha-adrenergic agonists are found to have effects on sleep. Its use for the control of hypertension in geriatric population is not preferred due to its effects on sleep and other CNS effects. Class I antiarrhythmics are known to be associated to cause somnolence or insomnia in some patients. Reduced sleep quality is reported by these patients. Sleep effects are also reported with use with Class IV antiarrhythmics in some individuals. Patients on ACE inhibitors, HMG CoA reductase, also report sleep problems at times. The effects on sleep are individually specific, and there is a need to carefully monitor sleep in these patients while on these drugs. Also, a careful choice of drug for patients who suffer from sleep problems is advisable to avoid further deterioration of sleep in these patients.

Endocrinal disorders affect sleep. Diabetes and associated hypoglycemia or hyperglycemia affect sleep. Sleep disorders can worsen glucose homeostasis. Nocturnal hypoglycemic episodes may be associated with nightmares, sweating profusely at night, spontaneous arousals, getting up crying or screaming, and confusional kind of arousals. Daytime sleepiness may be seen in cases of acromegaly. Insomnia may be associated with hyperthyroidism and menopause. Disrupted sleep is seen in Cushing's, pregnancy, and postpartum. The sleep disruption may be seen due to painful neuropathy in diabetes. Studies are reported showing increased association of sleep apnea with menopause, Cushing's, acromegaly, diabetes, and hypothyroidism. Reduced sleep continuity and sleep quality may be associated with reduced slow wave sleep in cases of Cushing's, Addison's disease, and hypothyroidism. Careful history taking and high suspicion are key for early diagnosis and management of these cases.

Overnight recording of sleep is reported for cardiac events specifically. The presence or absence of sinus bradycardia, tachycardia, asystole, wide and narrow complex tachycardia, atrial fibrillations, and other ectopic and altered rhythms or cardiac blocks must be reported in the polysomnography. Reporting of these events and their criteria is further dealt with in detail in Chapters 20 and 21 on polysomnography. The treating physician may correlate the presence of these findings with the bothering symptoms of the patient like palpitations, arousals, sweating, etc. at night.

Cardiovascular symptoms might also be seen in cases of seizure, and seizure might be triggered by an underlying cardiovascular pathology. Seizures may manifest as a cardiopulmonary cause, and vice versa also holds true. Often seizure may be confused with other disorders like periodic limb movement disorder, parasomnias, and recurrent arousals in insomnia. In sleep deprivation, sleep paralysis is seen, which can be often confused with postseizure states by caregivers. Seizure and panic attacks may also coexist. Commonly seen nonmotor symptoms in Parkinsonism are insomnia and altered sleep and vigilance. REM sleep behavior disorders, parasomnias, excessive daytime sleepiness, and narcolepsy-type complaints might show altered perception of time and abnormal sleep-wake transition, recurrent nightmares, and confusion in dream and reality. Lesions in the REM atonia system may also be seen.

An extended montage for seizure detection at night with continuous video monitoring is required to diagnose nocturnal seizures during sleep. In-attendance, continuous monitoring by a technician might be required since it is difficult to diagnose seizures on the record due to masking of the seizure activity by movement artifacts or the lack of it being picked up by scalp EEG electrodes. A seizure might mimic a sudden arousal, and therefore the night technician should diligently be in attendance throughout the patient monitoring and take detailed notes of all suspicious events.

Atrial fibrillation is a common association in stroke patients. Hypertension, atrial fibrillation, sleep disordered breathing, and transient ischemic attacks are known risk factors for stroke. Stroke patients may have various types of sleep complaints depending on the site and extent of lesion in the brain. Common sleep disorders seen are hypersomnia, obstructive sleep apnea, dream like hallucinations, and central apnea. Central sleep apnea and hypopnea may be seen with Cheyne-Stokes breathing probably due to CO_2 hypersensitivity induced by the lesion itself. Brain stem stroke might bring on central hypoventilation and other breathing problems. In thalamic and mesencephalic stroke, hypersomnia may be seen, and dream-like hallucinations may be associated with midbrain stroke. Sleep disordered breathing is found in almost 50% of stroke patients.

Even after addressing the obvious sleep problems, if the patient keeps on complaining of feeling "unfresh" despite having adequate opportunity to sleep, it may be a cause of concern. At this juncture, one must investigate for other coexisting sleep disorders that may affect the sleep quality of the patient.

Also, some undiagnosed comorbidities like concomitant hypertension, cardiac, or neurological pathology, diabetes, GERD, anxiety, mood disorders, etc. must be looked for. In patients who lack a bed partner, a history of witnessed apnea or snoring might be easily missed. The presence of witnessed apnea signifies periods of hypoxia during sleep. Hypoxia has its effects on the heart, kidney, brain, and vasculature all over the body. This may be the harbinger of the onset of many diseases and a reason for the deterioration caused by existing diseases.

Associated sleep breathing disorders, if suspected, require a workup using overnight recording, and assessment of the severity assists the management of these cases adequately. Disorders like corpulmonale and Cheyne–Stokes breathing may further aggravate the condition.

Sleep problems are also commonly associated with headaches. Migraine is found to be associated with sleep onset, or it might originate during deep sleep. Headaches might be present upon waking up, which may be commonly associated with obstructive sleep apnea, bruxism, depression, and hypertension. Masseter hypertrophy or worn-out teeth due to grinding, hint at the presence of bruxism.

Traumatic brain injury and spinal cord lesion patients might complain of multiple types of sleep problems like insomnia, hypersomnia, restless sleep, or even narcolepsy at times.

A history of recent head injury may be of value in patients having an unexplained onset of problems at work due to excessive sleepiness during the daytime. The subtle history of suboptimal performance during daytime due to excessive sleepiness should raise an alarm, and a detailed history taking to elicit possible causes should be done.

Patients with Alzheimer's dementia may complain of unrestorative sleep, and polysomnography might show reduced K-complexes and slow wave sleep. Periodic limb movement disorder, restless leg syndrome, and REM behavior disorder are also seen in these patients.

The bidirectional relationship of bad sleep and common disorders is an important factor that should be considered during practice. This is even more significant because the patients themselves do not pay attention to their sleep, and even if they have problems, they usually underestimate the effects of them.

CONCLUSION

At a primary care level, the early detection of common sleep problems like delayed sleep onset, poor sleep quality, poor maintenance of sleep, snoring, witnessed apnea, history of palpitations and sweating, sudden unexplained arousals, etc. may help the patient in the long run. Often, subtle sleep complaints might hint at underlying cardiovascular, neurological, or endocrinal and metabolic disorders. Knowledge of cardiovascular, endocrinal, and neurological disorders that might have associated sleep disorders is important to pick up.

11

Is There a Complaint of Depression, Anxiety, Stress, etc.?

DEEPAK SHRIVASTAVA

RELATIONSHIP BETWEEN SLEEP AND PSYCHIATRIC DISORDERS

The majority of psychiatric disorders are known to cause sleep disturbance. Nearly 30% of subjects with insomnia or excessive daytime sleepiness present some evidence of an underlying psychiatric disorder, most commonly related to anxiety and mood. A complex relationship between the sleep patterns and the psychiatric diseases is intermixed with a heightened state of arousal as well as anxiety. This combination worsens the mood disorders. Insomnia is well-known to precede by many months the clinical depression that is recognizable. Insomnia has a similar relationship with generalized anxiety disorder. Such an association further leads to alcohol and drug use and other maladaptive behaviors. In other words, it is safe to say that insomnia is predictive of an impending psychiatric condition.

MOOD DISORDERS

Sleep problems are commonly reported in primary care patients with mood disorders. These disorders include bipolar disorder manifested by manic, mixed hypomanic states and by major depressive disorder (MDD). Both these disorders have high rates of suicide.

Major Depressive Disorder

MDD is diagnosed based on depressed mood, loss of pleasure in activities of life, and loss of interest during episodes of MDD. Sleep abnormalities and specific patterns are common during the acute episodes of mood disorder. As noted, the most common symptom is disrupted sleep, as well as insomnia. Insomnia could be sleep onset insomnia, manifested by difficulty falling asleep, increased wake-up time during the major sleep period, and awakening earlier in the morning with daytime impairment secondary to nonrestorative sleep. Patients sometimes do not relate nighttime sleep problems with daytime tiredness and fatigue. Patients may report disturbing nightmares and dreams and a sense of less need for sleep especially in manic and hypomanic states. Patients with bipolar disorder tend to have seasonal affective

DOI: 10.1201/9781003093381-13

disorder and excessive need for sleep that could last up to 18–22 hours a day. There is difficulty in morning awakening and the need for continuous sleep and naps throughout the day.

Typical polysomnography findings demonstrate long sleep latency, increased wake time during the night, early morning awakening, poor sleep efficiency, and reduced total sleep time. There is a decreased percentage of N3 slow wave sleep. Both the depressive and the manic episodes cause significant impairment of family and social relationships, as well as impaired occupational functioning. In patients with mood disorder REM sleep, abnormalities have been noted: remarkable changes in the distribution and amount of REM sleep as well as a depressed patient's early onset of REM sleep (reduced REM latency) and an increase in phasic REM activity, increased duration of the first REM cycle, and increase in the total REM time throughout the night. In fact, many of patients more or less showed similar sleep abnormalities as described in depressed patients.

Treatment of the Major Mood Disorders Affecting Sleep

Mood disorders improved with antidepressant treatment. The newer antidepressants—including selective serotonin uptake inhibitors like paroxetine, sertraline, and fluoxetine, as well as serotonin and norepinephrine retyped inhibitors (SNRI), such as duloxetine and venlafaxine—are effective and have a better side effect and safety profile compared to tricyclic antidepressant or MAO inhibitors. These are considered the first-line therapy for depression. Bupropion is a commonly used medication in cases of depression. One has to be careful regarding the induction of insomnia in patients with this therapy.

Tricyclic antidepressants continue to have some control in the management of mood disorders affecting sleep. For patients with insomnia, due to the anticholinergic effect of tricyclic antidepressant causing increased sleepiness, tricyclics can be used. In general, their tolerance is poor due to the side effects of urinary retention, hypotension, blurred vision, and dry mouth. There is a risk of cardiac arrhythmias.

For patients who present with psychotic symptoms, several newer, very effective antipsychotic medications are available, among them olanzapine and quetiapine.

Most antidepressants have a significant effect on sleep architecture including increased REM latency, reduced percentage of REM sleep, and total REM sleep time

Lithium Carbonate

Lithium is a common mood stabilizer generally used to treat patients with bipolar disorder. Other drugs for bipolar disorder treatment are sodium valproate and carbamazepine. Mood stabilizers are sedatives but do not change sleep architecture. Lithium, however, can potentially increase N3 slow wave sleep and suppress REM sleep.

Nefazodone is a serotonin receptor antagonist and is considered a good-quality antidepressant with REM-sleep suppressing-effects. It decreases the total wake time and increases the percentage of N2 sleep. It does have a black box warning regarding liver toxicity.

A few medications, including nefazodone, bupropion, trimipramine, and trazodone, do not have any effect on REM sleep.

ANXIETY DISORDERS

Anxiety is one of the most common symptoms encountered in modern society. Generalized anxiety disorder is a psychiatric disease. Anxiety is related with insomnia and is a response to acute negative situations, causing stress response. Sleep study findings demonstrate increased sleep latency, frequent awakening, decreased sleep efficiency, and decreased amount of total sleep. Anxiety does not cause any change in REM sleep.

Generalized anxiety disorder (GAD) is a chronic and persistent form of anxiety. These patients are unable to fall asleep or maintain sleep. Most of the time, they complain of insomnia. Just like situational anxiety, also known as adjustment anxiety disorder, patients with GAD in sleep studies also showed problems with sleep maintenance and falling asleep. Total sleep time is decreased, and there are early morning awakenings.

Anxiety is most commonly managed with benzodiazepines taken at bedtime. Some patients are highly sensitive to the effects of benzodiazepine and may demonstrate excessive daytime sleepiness.

SSRIs and SNRI, as well as tricyclic antidepressants, have been used successfully in the management of GAD. These medications, while controlling anxiety, can worsen insomnia that should be treated with appropriate medication at nighttime. Excellent sleep hygiene and behavioral and relaxation therapies contribute to good-quality sleep.

PANIC ATTACK DISORDER

Typical panic disorder is the sudden onset of extreme anxiety along with associated shortness of breath, palpitation, high heart rate, choking sensation, severe chest pain, sweating, nausea and occasional vomiting, and trembling episodes of feeling of impending doom. Panic attacks can occur during both sleep and wakefulness. The sleep studies show a higher incidence of panic attacks during non-REM sleep in transition from Stage N2 to N3 sleep. Panic attacks can also occur in REM sleep. Panic attacks sometimes can be confused with sleep terrors. Patients suffer from insomnia due to the fear of precipitating another panic attack if they fall asleep. Benzodiazepines, including alprazolam and clonazepam, SSRI, and SNRI with tricyclic antidepressants are generally effective in controlling panic attacks.

POSTTRAUMATIC STRESS DISORDER (PTSD)

PTSD develops in patients who have experienced a traumatic event and now have flashbacks, recurring dreams of the event, as well as heightened arousal. Patients may present with complaints of nightmares, inability to fall asleep, or insomnia. Multiple abnormalities in the sleep study have been described in REM sleep as well as non-REM sleep. No patterns have been established. The close differential diagnosis includes panic attacks and night terrors. Insomnia may be the result of avoiding falling asleep to prevent the recurring experience. SSRIs are generally used to manage PTSD. While other medications like tiagabine, prazosin, and atypical antipsychotics have been tried; psychotherapy and cognitive behavioral therapy have been reportedly helpful.

OBSESSIVE-COMPULSIVE DISORDER (OCD)

Patients with obsessive-compulsive disorder have continuously decreased sleep and reduction in REM latency. These patients have intrusive thoughts, impulsive behavior, and repetitive tasks in order to reduce distress. Normal sleep onset is disturbed because of patient's thought process as well as obsessive-compulsive behavior. These patients are currently treated with SSRIs including fluoxetine, sertraline, and paroxetine as well as clomipramine and venlafaxine.

SCHIZOPHRENIA

Typical sleep-related symptoms in schizophrenia patients include problems with falling asleep and maintaining sleep through the night. They also sometimes have nightmares. The disrupted sleep results in daytime symptoms of tiredness and fatigue and the need for frequent napping. Sleep studies have shown increased sleep latency, poor and decreased sleep efficiency, as well as decreased total sleep time in patients with schizophrenia. REM sleep abnormalities include reduced REM sleep latency. Other changes are not consistent.

The mainstay of schizophrenia treatment is antipsychotic therapy with supportive care. Antipsychotic medications have significant side effects and intolerances. The newer antipsychotic medications clozapine and risperidone have a somewhat better side effect profile and appear to be more efficacious. Most antipsychotic medications have sedative effects. Clozapine increases total sleep time and sleep efficiency but decreases N3 slow wave sleep. Olanzapine improves sleep continuity and increases N3 slow wave sleep. Risperidone increases N3 slow wave sleep. Risperidone is less sedating compared to the other two newer antipsychotics. Patients with schizophrenia tend to have a higher incidence of narcolepsy, obstructive sleep apnea, and periodic limb movements.

12

Is the Patient a Child? Is the Patient Pregnant? Other Special Cases

DEEPAK SHRIVASTAVA

THE CHILD AS A SLEEP PATIENT

OSA and Narcolepsy

The major disorders of excessive somnolence in children are obstructive sleep apnea and narcolepsy.

Narcolepsy patients report that their symptoms began before age 15. Cataplexy is reported in only 50–70% of children. Cataplexy may be as subtle as twitching or weakness in the knees in response to emotional or other stimuli.

Insomnia in Children

Children sometimes won't sleep. At 3 years of age, 13% of children have problems settling, and 14% remain awake at night. The most important step in the evaluation of the sleepless child is obtaining a good-quality history. Although the parents often report the worst night experience, it is important to get an accurate description of the usual patterns. What does the child do in the evening before

bed, at bedtime, and during any night awakenings? What are the interactions with parents and other household members? What conditions must be present under which the child falls asleep or back to sleep? The sleeping environment should be explored. Who sleeps where, in a bed or crib, nighttime lighting, open or closed door, music, bottles, pacifiers, transitional objects?

Behavioral Insomnia of Childhood

Insomnia in children can generally be characterized as *sleep onset association disorders* and *limit-setting sleep disorders*. Brief awakenings at night are normal in children. Children who are used to falling asleep while they are being held, rocked, or patted may be unable to fall asleep unless those associations are repeated. When children who are usually rocked to sleep have a normal nighttime awakening, they find themselves in unfamiliar circumstances and are unable to get back to sleep. This results in crying or other undesirable behaviors until the parent recreates the setting wherein the children fell asleep.

Treatment of sleep onset association disorders involves educating the parent that night awakenings are normal, that sleep onset associations are simple habits, and that new sleep onset associations can be taught. Children must learn to fall asleep under the conditions they will find themselves in when they experience the normal nighttime awakenings, that is, alone and in their own bed or crib. The family is taught to maintain a constant, non-stressful bedtime ritual. A child is placed in his or her own bed or crib while awake, and the parent leaves the room. If the child is upset, the parent may return to the room after a few minutes and verbally comfort the child briefly, gradually increasing the time out of the room until the child falls asleep. The specifics can vary based on the individual family's circumstances. Children are very inventive. If one request does not work, they abandon it for another, but once they find one that is successful, they are sure to repeat it.

Parents must be educated that limit setting is a part of good parenting and not cruelty. They must decide in advance on the bedtime ritual and stick to it (e.g., one book, one glass of water). The child must consistently be returned to bed if he or she leaves the room; a gate may be necessary. Children usually respond well to positive reinforcement such as a star chart.

Childhood Parasomnias

Parasomnias are episodic disorders in sleep, rather than a disorder of wakefulness or sleep, per se. They usually do not produce a primary complaint of insomnia or excessive sleepiness.

Confusional Arousals

These events usually take place following arousals from sleep, most typically deep sleep in the first part of the night. Episodes may last several minutes. There is often absence of recollection of mental activity. They represent an admixture of wakefulness into non-REM sleep. Patients partially awaken and exhibit marked confusion, slow mentation, disorientation, perceptual impairment. The memory of the event is often absent. This type of arousal is commonly reported in children.

Predisposing factors to confusional arousals include any factors that induce deep sleep and impair the awakening threshold. Populations at risk are individuals who are sleep deprived, those who are recovering from sleep deprivation, and patients who are exposed to fever and CNS depressants. Confusional arousals are common under age 5 years and with increasing age become less common. The sex ratio is equal.

The differential diagnosis of confusional arousals includes sleep terrors, sleepwalking, REM behavior disorder and nocturnal epileptic seizures. There is a strong familial tendency for confusional arousals, and formal genetic studies are still pending.

Polysomnographic studies reveal abnormalities during the first one-third of the night and appear to be very rare during REM sleep. Confusional arousals are common during transition periods from non-REM to REM sleep. The EEG during confusions may show a brief episode of delta activity (SWS), stage 1 theta pattern, and repeated microsleeps.

Sleepwalking (Somnambulism)

Sleepwalking is a complex behavior that occurs during N3 sleep. It results in walking while asleep. Communication with the patient is often difficult. The behaviors may be of a wide range of a repetitive nature and have a symbolic meaning.

The risk of injury is a major concern in sleepwalking. Sleepwalking often lasts from 1 to 5 minutes, but, rarely, episodes may last more than an hour if behavioral spells are complex. Hybrid attacks may occur, during which time sleep terrors precede the sleepwalking and evolve into it.

Homicidal somnambulism is a parasomnia with considerable medicolegal implications. Predisposing factors may include several medications that can exacerbate or induce sleepwalking. Some of these include chloralhydrate, lithium, fluphenazine, perphenazine, and desipramine. Fevers can generally produce and increase the frequency of sleepwalking episodes. Other precipitants include CNS suppression, untreated obstructive sleep apnea, stress, and a distended bladder.

The prevalence of sleepwalking is 1–15% percent of the general population. The peak incidence is usually between the ages of 4 and 8, and sleepwalking incidents usually disappear spontaneously later in life.

The differential diagnosis includes nocturnal eating. These are episodes of awakening with the inability to return to sleep without eating or drinking. Other nocturnal spells on the differential diagnosis of sleepwalking include sleep-related partial complex seizures, RBD, confusional arousals, and episodic nocturnal wandering. The sex ratio is equal. Familial patterns are reported. The incidence of sleepwalking is 22% if neither parent suffers from a history of sleepwalking, 45% if only one parent is affected, and 60% if both parents are affected.

Polysomnographic features show that sleepwalking begins in N3 and appears more commonly at the end of the first or second episode of N3. EEG results demonstrate "lightning" from N3 into lighter sleep stages (N1 and N2). There is often a lack of autonomic activation. Delta bursts and an increase in microarousals may be observed. Polysomnographic monitoring is routinely done with video recording using a long cable.

Treatment is based on avoidance of precipitating factors and securing a safe home environment. This is accomplished by removing sharp, dangerous items from the bedroom, locking doors, using alarms, hiding car keys, and use of a bedroom downstairs. Tricyclic antidepressants and benzodiazepines have been used in refractory cases. Psychological and psychiatric treatment, together with reassurance, is needed when patients have a history of a psychological factor that prompts the appearance of these spells.

Sleep-Related Eating Disorders

Sleep-related eating disorders are recurrent episodes of eating during sleep without being aware of the activity. They often are associated with significant weight gain and are common in young women.

Sleep Terrors (*Pavor Nocturnus Incubus*)

Sleep terrors are a syndrome that consists of a sudden arousal associated with screaming or behavior related to being afraid and crying. The child cannot be woken up and does not have memory of the event in the morning.

Sleep terror is often an extreme autonomic arousal. Sleep terrors are associated with increased heart and respiratory rate, sweating, flushed skin, and muscle tone changes. Many times incoherent phonation or urinary incontinence can occur.

There may be a variable motor activity such as extreme agitation or escape behavior. These are states of cerebral hyperresponsiveness. The spells may be dangerous, as patients may hurt themselves during the escape behavior. There may be a sense of "oppression"; therefore, the name incubus (*in* = upon, *cubare* = to press upon). There were medieval beliefs that the attacks were prompted by a "devil" sitting or pressing on the chest of the sleeper. Sleep terrors usually last between half a minute to 3 minutes. Predisposing factors include forced awakening from N3, febrile illness, sleep deprivation, emotional stress, and CNS depressants, such as alcohol. Sleep terrors are prevalent in approximately 3% of children and 1% of adults, and men are more commonly affected than women. Psychopathology is rare in affected children but may have a stronger role in adult patients. Familial patterns show occurrence in several members of a single family.

The differential diagnosis of sleep terrors includes nightmares, anxiety attacks related to sleep disordered breathing, cardiac ischemia, and sleep-related epileptiform seizure activity.

Polysomnographic features demonstrate that the spells usually begin in SWS in the first third of the major sleep cycle. The events are accompanied by autonomic hyperarousal, as noted previously.

Treatment is often not required if episodes of sleep terrors are rare. For frequent episodes, short-acting benzodiazepines are recommended.

Rhythmic Movement Disorders

Rhythmic movement disorders (RMD) are manifested by repetitive, stereotyped rhythmic movements that involve the head and entire body. They may take the form of nocturnal head banging and body rocking or body rolling. The onset typically occurs within the first 2 years of life and may affect up to 20% of healthy children. Persistence into adulthood is rare and may be associated with significant psychopathological disorders, such as autism. The male-to-female ratio is approximately 3:1. Rare complications resulting from these movements, when very severe, may include skull callus, retinal petechiae, and subdural hemorrhage.

The diagnostic criteria for RMD include spells that occur during drowsiness or sleep and are accompanied by least one of the following:

- **Head banging:** The head forcibly moves in the anterior to posterior direction. The patient lies prone and repetitively lifts the head or the entire body, then "bangs" the head down into the pillow/mattress.
- **Head rolling:** The head moves sideways when the child is lying face up.
- **Body rocking:** The whole-body rocks when the child is in the knee-chest position. The entire body may roll forward and backward from a sitting position.
- **Body rolling:** The whole body is moved laterally (side to side) while in the supine position.

Video monitoring may reveal typical movements comprising rhythmic oscillation of the head and limbs. The rhythm frequency is between 0.5 to 2 Hz in long clusters with rhythmic "chanting" and other vocalization.

Head Banging

This is more likely to be present during REM sleep, while body rocking is more likely to be present during light sleep (stages N1 and N2). In the diagnostic workup of these episodes, one should assess for any underlying neurologic or psychiatric disorder that may cause the symptoms (i.e., nocturnal epilepsy).

The differential diagnosis includes bruxism, thumb sucking, PLMS, and infantile spasms. When adults manifest RMD, consideration should be given to neurologic or psychiatric causes.

Treatment is often not necessary. Parents may consider the use of bed padding and a protective helmet if the episodes lead to excessive noise or bodily injury. Behavioral modification may be used, and, if the episodes are severe, short-acting benzodiazepines or TCAs may be used. The parents also need to be reassured.

Nightmares

Ten to 50% of children aged 3–5 years, in general suffer with nightmares that disturb the parents. The polysomnogram may demonstrate increased blood pressure and sweating during the attack. Nightmares may occur during both non-REM and REM sleep. Non-REM nightmares are associated with pure fear without visual imagery, while REM nightmares are often vivid and frightening. There is an equal sex ratio in children.

Somniloquy (Sleep Talking)

Sleep talking is very common in children and usually of little concern to parents. It may be related to other parasomnias, such as sleepwalking, sleep terrors, and confusional arousals. It can occur in any stage of sleep.

SLEEP AND SLEEP DISORDERS DURING PREGNANCY

In women with preexisting sleep disorders, if taking medications, it is optimal to stop these medications prior to pregnancy and discontinue them once pregnancy begins.

If a woman has narcolepsy or idiopathic hypersomnolence, she should discontinue modafinil, methylphenidate, amphetamines, and other stimulants prior to becoming pregnant, if possible. Patients should be informed that once they stop taking their alerting medication, they should stop driving because of their increased risk of falling asleep while driving. Furthermore, they should assess their ability to stay alert for other important activities, including childcare and their job. Certain medications, like selective serotonin reuptake inhibitors and tricyclic antidepressants, do not cause major organ malformations; however, their use should be individualized. In women with depression, the decision to discontinue antidepressants should be made carefully by the physician and patient by examining the risk–benefit ratio.

In women who become pregnant with preexisting RLS, monitor iron, ferritin, vitamin B12, and folate levels, and supplement as tests indicate. Unfortunately, benzodiazepines, dopaminergic agents, and antiepileptic medications used to treat RLS are contraindicated in pregnancy. If severe symptoms are present, some professionals use opioids in this situation. However, opioids should be discontinued prior to delivery because of fetal respiratory depression.

In women with known sleep apnea, consider performing overnight pulse oximetry at intervals throughout the pregnancy, verifying adequate oxygenation during sleep. Because many women gain weight, their CPAP requirements may change during pregnancy. Of note, there are no data examining the use of automatic CPAP in this setting.

Check serum folate, vitamin B12, ferritin, iron, and hemoglobin early in pregnancy in all women, and supplement them if necessary. This has the potential to prevent RLS symptoms during the third trimester. Also, screen for snoring and OSA symptoms, especially in women with preeclampsia or in women who develop hypertension or proteinuria during their pregnancy.

Treatment of UARS or OSA with CPAP has the potential to improve fetal outcomes and hypertension, especially in preeclamptic women. Medication used for sleep disorders during pregnancy must be carefully evaluated, and the risk-benefit ratio must be considered for each.

Postpartum Sleep

After delivery, many women have sleep difficulties. Pain is present with both cesarean and vaginal deliveries. Infant feeding schedules interfere with sleep-wake schedules. The entire social environment of the mother is changed. Some women co-sleep with their infant, which may further disrupt their sleep. Multigravida mothers are better able to sleep than primigravida mothers in the postpartum period. Coble and colleagues noted that postpartum blues are experienced by 75–80% of women 3–5 days after giving birth, when there are hormonal changes. They noted a relationship between infant sleep disturbance and maternal

Table 12.1 FDA Pregnancy Category B Medications.

Antidepressant Medications
    Fluoxetine
    Paroxetine
Narcolepsy Medications
Hypnotic Medications
    Diphenhydramine
    Zolpidem
Gastroesophageal Reflux Medications
    Rabeprazole
    Esomeprazole
    Lansoprazole
    Pantoprazole
    Famotidine
    Cimetidine
    Ranitidine

mood depression. Postpartum depression and psychosis occur 2–4 weeks after childbirth and have a peak intensity 3–5 months postpartum. Two-thirds of women with postpartum depression do not have a prior history of depression. Most women have significant sleep deprivation postpartum, which improves 6–12 months later when the infant sleeps through the night.

Women are prone to many primary sleep disorders, including RLS, insomnia, fibromyalgia syndrome, and depression. There are also chronotherapeutic issues concerning women-associated cancers. Furthermore, women may be susceptible to collateral damage from a bed partner's or other family member's sleep disorders. The prevalence of OSA/SDB increases markedly around menopause.

RLS is more prevalent in women. Berger and colleagues performed a cross-sectional survey of 4310 participants (aged 20–79 years old) who were randomly selected from population registers. RLS was defined by the minimal criteria of the International Restless Legs Syndrome Study Group. The authors noted that RLS prevalence increased with age and affected 10.6% of the population. Furthermore, women were twice as likely as men to be affected. The prevalence of RLS in nulliparous women was like that in men. Parity was a major risk factor for developing RLS. For instance, women with one child had an increased odds ratio of 2.3 for developing RLS.

Menopause and Sleep

Menopause is fraught with hormonal, physiologic, and psychological changes that can lead to sleep disruption, including insomnia. Sleep complaints increase as women enter menopause and affect approximately 63% of menopausal women. Owens and Matthews reported the findings of a 3-year longitudinal study of healthy premenopausal women and characterized their sleep as they entered menopause. Women had difficulty falling asleep, had more nighttime awakenings, and woke up earlier than desired.

Major causes of sleep disruption during the perimenopausal and menopausal states include hot flashes, mood disorders, primary insomnia, and SDB. Addressing these causes has the potential to markedly improve sleep. Hot flashes disrupt sleep and affect up to 85% of perimenopausal and menopausal women. Approximately 25% of these women will experience hot flashes for more than 5 years.

Menopausal status also affects the likelihood of developing OSA/SDB, and menopause is an independent risk factor for SDB. Sleep apnea incidence was also influenced by the waist:hip ratio, which changes with female hormonal status.

Sleep architecture changes in menopause. There is a nonsignificant overall reduction in total sleep time with increased fragmentation of the sleep period. There are more arousals and more time awake with arousals.

13

Is the Patient Not Sleeping on Time?

KARUNA DATTA

INTRODUCTION

As we have seen in the previous chapters on the physiology of sleep and circadian rhythm, two important processes affect circadian rhythm and sleep. Process C regulates the circadian rhythm and is entrained by light-dark cycles, and Process S is regulated by the homeostatic need for sleep, which is directly proportional to the duration of wakefulness. The interaction of the two processes generally happens such that the individual sleeps the best at nighttime and is awake and alert during daytime. Any advancement or delay in the biorhythm of sleep-wake that desynchronizes with the light-dark cycle over a period may cause symptoms related to day and night dysfunction. Such a dysfunction that persists for a period of 3 months qualifies as a circadian rhythm sleep-wake disorder (CRSWD). This chapter discusses various types of CRSWD, their diagnosis, and management recommendations.

UNDERSTANDING THE UNDERLYING FACTORS AND THE PROBLEM

The problem of not being able to sleep at a habitual sleep time as per society norms, during the night, primarily might be due to two major reasons. First,

the problem can be intrinsically in the internal circadian rhythm and sleep drive referred to as intrinsic CRSWD. Second, it may be a problem of the external entrainment; i.e., light, social factors, or requirement of the individual to be awake are not meeting or matching the circadian requirement. In other words, a misalignment between the biological circadian rhythm and the requirement or feasibility of sleep at a particular time leads to the patient's not being able to sleep as per societal norms. This second type is referred to as extrinsic CRSWD.

Now let us recapitulate the important physiological factors required for entrainment of the biological circadian rhythm. (For further details on the physiology of circadian rhythm and important physiological factors, refer to Chapter 2.)

Physiological factors required for entrainment of biological rhythm are as follows:

- **Photic**: Exposure to light
- **Nonphotic**: Social cues like bedtime, meal time, time of exercise, group effects, etc.

The most important factor for entrainment of biological rhythm, or zeitgeber, is exposure to light. Evidence suggests that even ordinary room light is capable of shifting the circadian phase

DOI: 10.1201/9781003093381-15

response curve and suppression of melatonin. The phase response curve for circadian rhythm to exposure to light depends on the core body temperature (CBT). When the exposure to light occurs before the minimum CBT (CBT_{min}), it delays the cycle, and when it is presented after the CBT_{min}, it advances the cycle. Another factor that affects the effect of light exposure on the phase response curve is the intensity of light. The greater the intensity is, the greater is the effect. The circadian system in humans is found to be very sensitive to short wavelength blue light. But at bright intensity, both white light and blue light show similar effects probably due to photoreceptor saturation. Light avoidance also shows effects on circadian rhythm, and thus both exposure of light and strategic avoidance of light help in shifting the circadian phase.

To understand the likelihood of the occurrence of the CBT_{min}, it is important to know the biological night for the individual. The CBT_{min} usually happens 2–3 hours before the wake-up time. In a normal setting, when the individual is sleeping at night and waking up early in the morning. The CBT_{min} is likely to happen 2–3 hours before early morning, which may be approximately 4–5 a.m. depending on the wake-up time of 7–8 a.m. In patients with extremely delayed sleep cycles, for example, for a patient sleeping at 3 a.m. and waking up at 1 p.m., it is likely that the CBT_{min} occurs at around 10–11 a.m. In such cases, if a light exposure is given during daytime in the morning at around 8–9 am considering it as daytime, it will cause further damage by delaying the sleep cycle since it is biologically nighttime for these patients. Hence complete history taking and understanding the patient's sleep-wake schedules are extremely important to entrain the biological rhythm.

Subtle placement of physiological and social cues can also help entrain the sleep-wake rhythm once we know our patient well enough. These methods can use social cues, bedtime, mealtime, time of exercise, etc. Over a period of time, especially in adolescents, it has been found that procrastination of sleep delays their circadian rhythm further, which is over and above the slight physiological delay seen in adolescence. Moreover, peer pressure to be on social media late at night, the habit of playing video games, watching movies late at night also affect the rhythm by the sensitivity of the biological clock to shorter wavelengths. Physical exercise too close to bedtime delays the rhythm.

Melatonin has a phase response curve that is 180° out of phase with the phase response curve of light exposure. Exogenous melatonin in the afternoon or early evening advances the circadian phase, and a morning dose can delay the phase.

GENERAL FEATURES OF CRSWD

These disorders occur due to the problem in the timekeeping by the biological circadian clock or due to its entrainment by photic and nonphotic stimuli. It can also happen due to the change in the light-dark cycle of the individual and the misalignment with the biological clock, which continues. As per the *International Classification of Sleep Disorders* (ICSD-3), this disruption of circadian rhythm pattern could be chronic or recurrent leading to sleep-wake disturbances like insomnia or excessive daytime sleepiness. These sleep-wake disturbances should cause clinically significant distress and impairment in the individual's performance.

CRSWD is divided into two broad categories: intrinsic and extrinsic.

Intrinsic CRSWD

- Delayed sleep-wake phase disorder
- Advanced sleep-wake phase disorder
- Non 24-hour sleep-wake rhythm disorder
- Irregular sleep-wake rhythm disorder

Extrinsic CRSWD

- Shift work
- Jet lag disorder

Assessment of the circadian rhythm can be done by subjective and objective methods. Subjectively, sleep logs, questionnaires like Horne Ostberg, Munich chronotype, children's chronotype, can be used. Objectively, actigraphy can be used to monitor the light-dark cycle and the patient's activity. Core body temperature and salivary melatonin levels can be assessed over the 24 hours, only if feasible.

Clinically, the aim of the assessment of the circadian rhythm is to understand:

- Sleep-wake behavior
- Light exposure times and duration
- Circadian phase position using CBT_{min}

- Determining dim light melatonin onset and melatonin rhythm, if feasible
- Determining cortisol rhythm, if feasible
- Evaluating daytime dysfunction—daytime sleepiness, mood alterations, etc.
- Fatigue or performance deficits

Some of the commonly seen CRSWD—delayed sleep-wake phase disorder, advanced sleep-wake phase disorder, shift work, and jet lag disorder—are discussed next.

DELAYED SLEEP-WAKE PHASE DISORDER (DSWPD)

DSWPD is a type of intrinsic CRSWD. It is characterized by a sleep onset and a wake time delayed by usually more than 2 hours (commonly seen may be a delay of 3–6 hours) as compared to the societal average norms. Some habits are commonly noticed in these patients like a habit of bedtime alcohol, history of sedatives, probably because the patient attempts to help improve sleep onset. These patients when asked to sleep continuously usually get up very late in the morning or almost in the afternoon. Hence if a sleep hygiene principle of waking up early morning at the same time is tried on them or if regularizing their morning wake-up time is tried, it may prove to be detrimental because it would lead to acute sleep deprivation, and the patient will complain of extreme sleepiness during daytime, irritability, and, sometimes in chronic cases, depression, mood and personality disorders, and reduced scholastic performance. These patients are usually seen to combat their sleepiness at daytime by indulging in excessive use of caffeine.

As per the *ICSD*-3 guidelines, the following criteria are used for diagnosing DSWPD:

- Symptoms must be present for a minimum of 3 months.
- The individual should have improvement in sleep quality when allowed to sleep ad libitum and demonstrate a consistent delayed sleep-wake 24-hour pattern. This delay can be demonstrated using sleep diary, sleep logs preferably using actigraphy if possible. This should be done for preferably 14 days.
- Lastly, the problem in sleep should not be due to any other sleep disorder, medical, neurological or mental disorder, or medication or substance abuse.

The pathophysiology of this disorder may range from a hypersensitive suppression of melatonin by light to the effect on light entrainment capability, or it may be associated with some genetic alterations related to the molecular basis of circadian rhythm generation, such as, PER3 gene alterations. DSPD is also seen at extreme latitudes where light exposure is compromised. It is also found after minor brain injury.

The diagnosis of these patients requires the problem to persist for 3 months or more and should have added daytime problems for this period of time. During the clinical interview, caregiver input is necessary, especially if the case is a child, adolescent, or a patient with brain injury.

The diagnosis is made by:

- Sleep logs/sleep diaries for a minimum of 1 week, preferably for 2 weeks.
- Questionnaires—Horne-Ostberg Morningness Eveningness Questionnaire, Munich Chronotype Questionnaire, or Sleep Timing Questionnaire. These are not confirmatory for diagnosis but show a predilection toward evening type in these patients.
- An actigraphy, if available, may be done for a minimum of 7 days (preferably for 14 days) to ascertain the diagnosis.
- Polysomnography is indicated only to rule out other sleep disorders that may be responsible for excessive daytime sleepiness and/or insomnia. DSWPD is commonly diagnosed in patients presenting with insomnia complaints. Polysomnography in these cases often shows a delayed sleep onset latency and a delayed REM onset latency during the conventional night. The patient has problems sleeping at a conventional sleep time. Despite the sleep quality being normal when woken up at a conventional wake-up time, patient show an inability to wake up, irritability, and inability to perform cognitive tasks in the morning. They also complain of reduced alertness and excessive sleepiness. These patients, when forced to sleep at conventional sleep times, complain of the inability to sleep and hence present to sleep clinics with insomnia symptoms. When allowed to sleep without waking up in the morning, the patient sleeps with a normal sleep quality for a single stretch duration, which is normal compared to average norms.

- It is important to rule out other medical or psychiatric causes: for example, affective disorders, insomnia, mood and personality disorders. It is also important to rule out other causes for excessive daytime sleepiness in cases where the sleep quality is reported to be low: for example, obstructive sleep apnea, center sleep apnea, restless leg syndrome, bruxism, nocturnal epilepsy, sleep-associated epileptic episodes, etc.

The goal of management in these cases is to align the circadian rhythm to the 24-hour light day cycle, ensuring good sleep hygiene and management of comorbid sleep disorders and psychiatric disorders, if any. Many types of strategies or combinations of these can be used in these patients depending on the response by the patients. Sleep-wake schedule prescription can be given in which the cycle can be set by chronotherapy, i.e., advancing sleep by 1–2 hours over 5–6 days and then again by 1–2 hours over a week until a desired sleep time is achieved. Going slow by an advancement of only 10–15 min per day to achieve the target of 1–2 hours over 5–6 days is found to be more patient compliant. This has to be accompanied by the principles of sleep hygiene, i.e., not smoking just before sleep time, not doing intense exercise before sleep time, strategically avoiding light during the late evening as per the prescription, keeping free of ambience noise during sleep time as advised, etc. Timed physical exercise can be added to help align circadian rhythm to the light-dark circle.

Avoidance of light at night-time can be prescribed as treatment to be followed, along with timed light therapy depending on the CBT_{min} expected to be taken. Light therapy of 2500 lux for 2 hours in the biological morning and light restriction in the evening have been reported in studies to advance phase by 1.4 hours. In delayed sleep-wake phase syndrome, 250 lux for 2 hours can be given in the biological morning. Thirty minutes of 10,000 lux has also been tried. Naturalistic dawn can be created with 250 lux of light intensity.

Light therapy may not be tolerated by all patients, especially those having photosensitivity or patients with eye diseases. Retinopathy is an absolute contraindication for bright light therapy. Patients may also report headaches after light therapy. Constant supervision should be done of patients, and consultation of ophthalmologists or dermatologists may be considered before starting therapy. Details about light therapy are given in Chapter 22.

Promotion of sleep by sedatives, especially by preponing the phase, may be tried. However, one must watch carefully for side effects the next day after waking up; sleepiness and the inability to stay alert may continue the next day. AASM does not recommend sleep-promoting drugs for the elderly with dementia in irregular sleep-wake disorder, another type of CRSWD. In case the diagnosis of DSWPD is not ascertained and only suspected, it may be best to avoid them.

Melatonin agonist at the biological evening may advance sleep. To advance sleep, 0.3 mg of melatonin is considered good enough. Melatonin alone is a very weak therapeutic agent for DSPD and requires care during its administration for its potential side effects. Some studies in children have reported combination therapy using melatonin, avoidance of light at biological nighttime, behavioral treatment to improve sleep hygiene, and postawakening light exposure in DSPD patients. Behavioral interventions of avoiding late night parties or habits that can delay sleep should be followed. Contraindications to melatonin include young children. Anticlotting drugs and medications for asthma have drug interactions with melatonin and hence should be avoided in patients on these drugs. Patients who drive regularly or operate heavy machinery are also advised not to take the drug. Pregnant women or those expecting to be pregnant should avoid melatonin. For further details on the side effects and contraindications, see chapter 24 on the pharmacological therapy of sleep disorders.

Various therapeutic options are available, and the treatment of DSWPD is challenging. Certain recommendations of AASM include timed melatonin or agonists for adults with or without depression, children, and adolescents with no other comorbidities, except with psychiatric comorbidities in which it is recommended too. Postawakening light exposure and multicomponent behavioral intervention is also recommended by AASM for children and adolescents.

A combination therapy using behavioral treatment using natural light exposure in the morning, following sleep hygiene principles and postawakening light therapy has been found to benefit adults and children suffering from delayed sleep phase syndrome.

Treatment of DSPD in children and adolescents is a challenge, and prevention is always better than a cure. It is important to identify these cases earlier and to advise parents and children to take adequate prevention measures before developing a severe disorder. Awareness among high school students is considered an effective strategy because self-discipline is the best form of ensuring prevention of these disorders.

ADVANCED SLEEP-WAKE PHASE DISORDER (ASWPD)

ASWPD is also a type of intrinsic CRSWD.

According to *ICSD*-3, ASWPD is characterized by:

- Advancement in sleep time and wake-up time, which is typically more than 2 hours as compared to the conventional societal norms;
- Symptoms that last for at least 3 months; and
- Unattributable to any other sleep disorder or any coexisting mental, neurological, medical disorder or any medication or substance abuse. The advancement in the phase should be demonstrable in sleep logs or preferably in actigraphy recording for a minimum of 7 days, preferably for 14 days.

Usually, these patients are elderly. In the elderly, a well-timed short nap in the early afternoon might help their productivity in the evening. In ASWPD, it is important to ask that the patient is not too tired by evening. This may be important as sometimes the ASWPD patient might have a preponderance to make errors by late evening due to prolonged wakefulness. A short nap is highly recommended for such cases.

A diagnosis of ASWPD is done by sleep logs or diaries, or by actigraphy if available. Polysomnography is indicated only if it is required to rule out other sleep disorders and medical, neurological, or psychiatric causes. In case the patient is young, it is extremely important to rule out other causes of increased somnolence in the evening time.

Delaying sleep by 1 hour a day or even half an hour per day so as to achieve a delay may be tried. Bright light exposure during the evening helps these cases. In advanced sleep phase syndrome, a biological evening exposure of 250 lux for 2 nights has been found to be useful. AASM has recommended the use of timed light therapy in adults as studies have reported improvement with light therapy in these cases vs. no therapy. For more details on the rationale, methods of light therapy, indications, and contraindications, please read Chapter 22.

SHIFT WORK DISORDER

Shift work disorder is an extrinsic CRSWD. This disorder is associated with shift work and in some cases persists even after the shift rotations are over. A reduction in total sleep time is seen with the report of insomnia and/or daytime sleepiness usually due to a recurring work schedule that overlaps the sleep time.

As per the *ICSD*-3, a diagnosis of shift work disorder can be done using the following:

- The symptoms are associated with a shift work schedule for at least 3 months and should not be attributable to any other sleep disorder or any other coexisting mental, neurological, medical disorder or any medication or substance abuse.
- The disruption should be demonstrable in sleep logs or preferably in actigraphy recording for a minimum of 7 days, preferably for 14 days.

The pathophysiology of shift work disorder is the difference in the ability to adapt between sleep-wake behavior and circadian physiology. In early morning shift workers, due to sleep inertia and inadequate opportunity to sleep, automobile accidents are very prevalent. Similar is the case for night shift workers. During the early morning hours of work, they have an irresistible urge to sleep if the sleep debt is not recovered before the duty. Rotating shifts, both counterclockwise and clockwise, have a problem. Rapid changes, i.e., multiple shifts per week, are more troublesome than slower changes of schedule.

It is important that they get adequate sleep despite the shift work. Proper sleeping conditions at home should be available after the shift.

Usually, two types of problems are seen. One is related to sleep, which can be insomnia and/or sleepiness, and the other is reduced alertness at the time of work or during waking hours, increasing the chance of errors and accidents. With timed light exposure using artificial means, one can phase advance or phase delay. Occupational adjustments ensuring light exposure during work hours and scheduled sleep during rest hours using a conducive room environment and ambience to sleep helps the worker. Dark goggles can be used by night shift workers to avoid the bright light exposure in morning when returning from work in the morning. A small nap before the night shift can further enhance cognitive performance and alertness. Avoiding tea and coffee during daytime and having some at night helps during a night shift. Depending on the time of the shift, light exposure can be planned.

Shift workers should undergo regular physical examination to check for:

- Early signs of increased fatigue, the sleep problems of excessive sleepiness during the time of work, or the inability to sleep at the time to sleep. In case fatigue and sleep problems are found, the health attendant and the physician must educate the individual along with his family to help shift worker prioritize to obtain adequate sleep. The need for "protected time" for sleep should be explained to the worker so that he or she gives due importance to it.
- Any cardiovascular history or recent onset of cardiovascular complaints.
- Sleep hygiene practice based on the shift. This is extremely important for safety at the workplace and for workers' health. Workers should be instructed to follow the protected sleep time: going to bed early in case of an early morning shift; using earplugs, white noise, switching off phones to help sleep; a darkened bedroom after shifts. A caffeine prescription may be given to avoid drowsiness during travel to work or at work. Use of dark glasses after a night shift can help avoid light exposure in the morning while getting back from work.
- Poor diet, use of nicotine, alcohol consumption, etc. exacerbate the shift work disorder. Early identification and educational awareness of the employee are needed.

Administratively, the number of shift changes should be slower over 3–4 weeks rather than a rapid change in the shift time. The employer can look after the needs of night shift employee, who require daytime facilities, e.g., banking at night, and other requirements.

JET LAG DISORDER

This disorder is an extrinsic CRSWD and is associated with transmeridian jet travel, usually across two or more time zones. According to *ICSD*-3 criteria, associated daytime dysfunction occurs within 1–2 days of travel. It is diagnosed as jet lag disorder only when it is not attributable to any other sleep disorder or any other coexisting mental, neurological, medical disorder or any medication or substance abuse.

Eastward travel is more difficult to adjust than westward travel. Pre-flight conditioning helps the passenger avoid jet lag disorder, for example, starting to wake up early in eastward flights. Circadian prescriptions can be made for susceptible individuals. Circadian prescriptions also help in sportspersons or when attending business meetings where one cannot afford a dip in performance upon arrival to the new location. Timed light and melatonin agonists can be tried to set or reset the light-dark cycles.

Basic points to be kept in mind for a circadian prescriptions before travel are as follows:

- Knowledge of the flight schedule—list the travel start date and time, landing date and time, the stopover's location and time duration.
- Determine the CBT_{min} using the habitual wake-up time
- Calculate the time difference between the existing location and the destination.
- Note the sunrise and sunset times of both places during the travel period.
- Determine the direction of travel:
  - Westward phase delay: The delay in pre-flight should never be more than 2 hours/day.
  - Eastward: Advance only with a maximum 7 hour difference; otherwise delay.
  - A preflight shift of 1 hour/day advance in sleep time may be considered for eastward travel, never more than 1.5 hours for advancing sleep. Also, advancing should be done only if the phase difference is of 7 hours in eastward travel; otherwise follow preflight delay in order to synchronize faster.
- Note the timed light exposure. The phase response curve is most sensitive 4 hours before and after the CBT_{min}.

- Timed melatonin (0.5 mg melatonin 4.5–5 hours before the usual sleep onset can advance the cycle).
  - The entire prescription can be prepared for preflight, during flight, and after landing to minimize the onset of jet lag disorder. Intermittent bright light exposures, wearing orange glasses to block blue spectrum, meal timings and sleep timings, and caffeine intake can be planned for the individual.
  - If the jet lag persists even after 2 weeks of travel, consider evaluation for psychophysiological insomnia.

Some things need to be kept in mind while prescribing timed light therapy. Light therapy may pose problem in cases with a history of photosensitive medications: for example, drugs like phenothiazines, antimalarials, psoralen, anticlotting drugs, etc. Retinopathy is an absolute contraindication for bright light therapy. Also, bright light therapy may not be acceptable for patients with eye diseases, and some have light-therapy-related headaches. The clinician is advised to monitor the patient on bright light therapy for side effects, and clinical discretion should be used. Ophthalmologists' and dermatologists' opinions should be taken prior to starting light therapy. For more details on the rationale, methods of light therapy, indications, and contraindications, see Chapter 22.

SUGGESTED READING

1. Auger RR, Burgess HJ, Emens JS, Deriy LV, Thomas SM, Sharkey KM. Clinical practice guideline for the treatment of intrinsic circadian rhythm sleep-wake disorders: advanced sleep-wake phase disorder (ASWPD), delayed sleep-wake phase disorder (DSWPD), non-24-hour sleep-wake rhythm disorder (N24SWD), and irregular sleep-wake rhythm disorder (ISWRD). An update for 2015. *J Clin Sleep Med.* 2015;11(10):1199–1236.

2. Smith MT, McCrae CS, Cheung J, Martin JL, Harrod CG, Heald JL, Carden KA. Use of actigraphy for the evaluation of sleep disorders and circadian rhythm sleep-wake disorders: an American Academy of Sleep Medicine clinical practice guideline. *J Clin Sleep Med.* 2018;14(7):1231–1237.

3. Dodson ER, Zee PC. Therapeutics for circadian rhythm sleep disorders. *Sleep Med Clin.* 2010;5(4):701–715. http://doi.org/10.1016/j.jsmc.2010.08.001.

4. Eastman CI, Burgess HJ. How to travel the world without jet lag. *Sleep Med Clin.* 2009;4(2):241–255. http://doi.org/10.1016/j.jsmc.2009.02.006.

14

Broad Approach to Common Case Scenarios with Complaints of Sleep

KARUNA DATTA

INTRODUCTION

After having seen various disorders in this section, this chapter discusses the broad frameworks in which the findings of the patient broadly fall. The common scenarios built in this chapter may present in a patient as a single form or in combinations of two or more of them. The case picture may also be seen in association with other common diseases like hypertension, diabetes, stroke, depression, stress conditions, etc. After a detailed interview and examination, if a patient has sleep complaints, these common presentations give an idea to the treating primary care physician as to which of them broadly fit the patient. The chapter also lays out some primary factors or certain symptoms about which one must find out in detail when a patient complains of sleep problems. In the end, an algorithm for a patient with excessive daytime sleepiness has been provided to help the physician when such a patient is encountered.

COMMON CASE SCENARIOS

Certain common scenarios are related to sleep complaints, which may be identified in outpatients or admitted patients with sleep complaints. The scenarios developed here are typically for an average adult and do not include the special conditions of a child, pregnancy, or a geriatric patient/adult with medical or surgical complications. These special conditions have been dealt with separately in other chapters; however, these scenarios may be present in these special conditions too. The scenarios are developed predominantly for educational purposes, and therefore the real-life case might have only partial resemblance or may be a combination of two or more of them. The aim of broadly categorizing them may be useful in clarifying your approach for clinical decision making and future referral and management.

Scenario 1

The patient is sleeping at nighttime regularly on time and waking up at a regular time most days, but it takes almost 30 minutes or more to get to sleep after going to bed to sleep. For example, bedtime is 10 p.m., wake-up time is 6 a.m., and sleep onset latency (SOL) is more than 30 minutes for at least 3 days of the week.

DOI: 10.1201/9781003093381-16

Ask for the frequency of this problem of increased SOL. Ask the patient for any daytime consequences, like reduced attention, alertness, or increased sleepiness during daytime, mood swings, dips in performance, etc. Ask the patient to write a sleep diary for preferably 14 days. Details on the sleep diary are available in Chapter 17. Upon analyzing the sleep diary, if it is found that the problem of not able to sleep after lying in bed for more than 30 minutes occurs more than 3 times a week, with daytime consequences, then as per the ICSD-3 criteria, the patient would be diagnosed as a case of insomnia. The duration of illness of more than 3 months can be categorized as chronic insomnia. Sometimes patients have this problem in episodes often associated with identifiable precipitating factors and spans over several years. It can be considered chronic insomnia. A detailed discussion on insomnia is available in Chapter 6. A similar scenario also categorized as insomnia is when the patient lies down to sleep regularly at bedtime, the onset of sleep is within minutes, but the patient wakes up during the night and is not able to sleep for almost 30 minutes or wakes up many times at night and the total wake time after sleep onset (WASO) may be more than 30 minutes. Another situation also categorized as insomnia is when the patient wakes up in the wee hours of the morning and just cannot sleep right up to the usual wake-up time and so finally gets out of the bed. All three of these situations are types of insomnia: sleep onset, sleep maintenance, and sleep termination. In a patient, all three types may be seen intermingled with one another over the course of weeks.

WASO is the amount of time awake after sleep onset and before wake-up. This time is affected by sleep breaks and hence is increased when the patient has frequent awakenings during the night after initially dozing off to sleep and before finally waking up. WASO may be calculated by the total duration of sleep breaks during the night. It may be objectively calculated using a polysomnography record or subjectively using a sleep diary. Details on the sleep diary, actigraphy, and polysomnography are given in Chapters 17, 18, 20, and 21)

Scenario 2

This patient complains of not feeling fresh throughout the day. The patient might complain about a slightly cloudy thought process and feels that decision making is slightly delayed. His or her normal bedtime might be late in the night or early morning, like at 2 a.m. or so. The patient says that there is no problem in falling off to sleep, in fact, falls asleep almost instantaneously and wakes up latest by 7 a.m. The usual reasons for the delayed bedtime are to complete office work, social commitments, and so on and hence the tendency to go to bed late. After waking up, the patient is not fresh in the morning and starts feeling better only after the morning coffee or tea. Sometimes these patients would have devised their own methods to make themselves alert after waking up. A requirement of tea or coffee, washing their face, etc. to ensure alertness might be their routine. Complaints of tardiness at work are also common, and they improve as the day progresses. Sometimes this behavior of sleeping late regularly and getting up early to meet the day's requirement is so chronic that the patient just gets used to it and might not even complain at all. Only upon detailed history taking might it come out.

Upon history taking, it will be clear that the patient does not provide enough opportunity to sleep, and this therefore falls into the category of sleep deprivation. Schoolchildren might be seen to work or play or to become distracted on social media until late at night and then have to get up to attend classes, thereby falling into a typical chronic sleep deprivation model. To further add to this practice, in adolescents, an additional feature of delayed circadian rhythm due to the hormonal changes during adolescence further aggravates the deprivation.

Scenario 3

This may be taken as a case where the individual sleeps very late at night and gets up very late in the morning: for example, bedtime 2 a.m. and wake-up time of 11 a.m. The patient has a history of falling off to sleep immediately once in bed to sleep. This pattern is seen commonly in college students. The problem starts when it becomes chronic. Lack of parental control on sleep timings in high school children might also result in this scenario. Weight gain, a dip in academic performance, social withdrawal, feeling unwell, having depressed thoughts, mood swings, and many other psychological problems may be present. This is how a delayed sleep-wake phase disorders that are a kind of circadian rhythm disorder would look like. Circadian rhythm disorders have been discussed in detail in Chapter 13.

Scenario 4

This may be slightly more complex than scenario 2. Here, the patient is not only late in sleeping and wakes up early due to commitments but takes also almost 30 minutes to sleep after deciding to sleep, unlike scenario 2, where the latency to go off to sleep after lying in bed to sleep was negligible. This patient definitely has effects of sleep deprivation but harbors insomnia in addition.

Scenario 5

This patient complains of unrefreshed sleep despite a regular bedtime at 10 p.m. and a wake-up time at 6 a.m. The patient drops off almost immediately after going to bed to sleep but still complains of not feeling fresh after getting up in the morning from a full night's sleep.

This patient needs to be investigated to find the cause for the unrefreshed sleep. Whatever the cause may be, either it is causing frequent arousals or is not letting the patient sleep deeply, hence deteriorating the sleep quality.

- It may be that the patient is snoring, with or without spells of apnea, which causes hypoxia and frequent awakening.
- There may be an association of movement disorders during sleep, which might be primarily a sleep problem: for example, periodic limb movement disorder during sleep, NREM or REM parasomnias. The movement disorders may also be due to neurological etiology of epilepsy, stroke, or conditions like Parkinson's disease commonly found associated with movement disorders.
- The cause of reduced sleep quality may be also due to substance abuse, cardiovascular etiology, stroke, GERD, laryngopharyngeal reflux disease, etc.
- Look for sleep disorders like bruxism, narcolepsy, or medical conditions that may affect the patient's sleep quality in this case.

Hence these patients may be harboring a disease that may be directly or indirectly the cause for impaired sleep quality. If the condition is severe or is associated with two or more conditions, we might find frequent awakenings at night. This patient, if left untreated and if the frequent awakenings at night are not managed, may also end up developing sleep maintenance insomnia (explained in scenario 1).

Scenario 6

This patient, a typical elderly patient complaining of waking up too early in the night, e.g., a wake-up time of 3 a.m. History taking reveals that the patient sleeps very early usually like 8 p.m. and then gets up at 3 a.m., after which there is a problem of not being able to sleep even after trying. So, the patient wakes up and starts the day very early. Upon questioning, the patient complains of an irresistible urge to go off to sleep after late evening, might also give a history of napping in the late evening, or making subtle errors owing to the sleepiness; gives history of not wanting to attend parties or social gatherings because of this irresistible urge to sleep much earlier than others. This patient has been able to sleep a good duration of 7 hours, but the entire phase of sleep time is preponed and hence is more likely to be an advanced sleep-wake circadian rhythm disorder, a type of circadian rhythm disorder, details of which are already discussed in Chapter 13. This case should not be confused with sleep termination insomnia, wherein the sleep abruptly ends in the middle of the night, and the patient is not able to go off to sleep again. In the case of sleep termination insomnia, bedtime was not earlier as in this case, and the duration of sleep is much less: for example, sleeping at 11 p.m. and waking up at 3 a.m. and then not being able to sleep, where the duration of sleep is much reduced. In scenario 6, however, the problem was not sleep duration but the timing of sleep, which was much earlier than society norms.

These scenarios are oversimplified for better understanding of the concept, but in real practice, we might see a combination of causes leading to the sleep complaint. As a health care worker, whether a physician or otherwise, it is important to understand the causes and address them. Hyperthyroidism may cause an inability to sleep, and not being able to sleep due to sudden onset headaches might be a red flag sign for a developing neurological cause. Lack of sleep quality may be due to frequent palpitations at night due to ectopic or coronary insufficiency. Frequent arousals might also be due to OSA, hypertension, chronic pain conditions, etc. This list is not complete, but these examples are mentioned just to highlight the need to take good history to identify the cause of the sleep problem.

SOME FACTORS AND SYMPTOMS TO KEEP IN MIND

While dealing with sleep complaints, some primary factors, symptoms, and presentations should be kept in mind:

- **Duration of sleep complaints:** If a clear-cut history of the duration is available, it makes the recording easier and faster, but often the complaints are so interwoven with other complaints and incidents in a patient's life that to elicit a clear-cut history of duration of sleep becomes difficult. At these times, one may start with asking the patient to go back in time by memory and think of a time when sleep was deep, refreshing and one felt like having slept "like a log." Such questions sometimes get very startling responses and might take the history back by decades. Once the starting point is identified, it may be easier to pinpoint the various incidents, causes, or associations that the patient remembers in reaching the present state. Once the duration is ascertained, it might be clear whether it is a continuous or episodic sleep complaint. For example, not being able to sleep after lying in bed might be associated with family stressors for a given patient and between the stressors, the patient might be feeling completely fine. On the other hand, another patient might have seen a slow steady deterioration over a period exaggerated with family stressors. The two presentations thus become different.

- **Duration of opportunity to sleep:** What amount of time does the patient assign to sleep? This necessarily may not be the amount of time the patient spends in bed. Many patients, especially adolescents and college students, would report that they are in bed from 11 p.m. to 7 a.m. But when further probed, they may admit that the opportunity given for sleep may be very less. This might be because of playing games or doing assignments/studying while in bed and other sleep hygiene issues. This may also direct us to some individual

nuances that might be required to be taken care off to improve the patient's sleep.

- **Predominant timing of sleep:** Is most of the sleep at night or during the daytime? Does the patient have one major bout of sleep or sleeps in small chunks throughout the day? Sometimes it may be found that the patient may be taking 2–3 major chunks of sleep. One natural sleep at night might be short due to sleep deprivation, and hence there may be a need for another big chunk during the afternoon. Also, a worktime shift to nighttime or to late evening may be responsible for such a state. Therefore, this history tells us about the regularity of the predominant timing of sleep. It may be beneficial to understand circadian rhythm disorders if present in the patient.

- **Sleep quality:** By sleep quality, what one wants to understand is the depth of sleep, i.e., whether the transitions from NREM and REM and from REM to NREM are smooth. The slow wave sleep quality and duration are both important for sleep quality and may be important for the feeling of being refreshed after sleep. Similarly, if the transitions from NREM to REM and REM to NREM sleep are without arousals, awakenings, or frequent posture shifts, the person might feel better. Clearly pinpointing what determines sleep quality is difficult and is a matter of scientific discussion, but, briefly, sleep that has adequate quality and duration of slow wave sleep and is free from interruptions may broadly be responsible for good sleep quality. Disorders that increase the sympathetic drive, increase physiological arousal, or lead to a presleep arousal state may also affect sleep quality. A detailed history on the perception of the patient's sleep quality might give an important clue to facilitate an early diagnosis of hypertension, diabetes, endocrinal disorders, parasomnias, ectopic rhythms, angina during sleep, GERD, other cardiovascular, neurological, psychological disorders, etc.

- **History of snoring with or without witnessed apnea, abnormal movements, and behavior:** This history may be elicited by a bed partner, caretaker, or a roommate who is awake or gets up to witness the person having apnea during sleep. Sometimes bed partners mention the history of witnessing abnormal movements

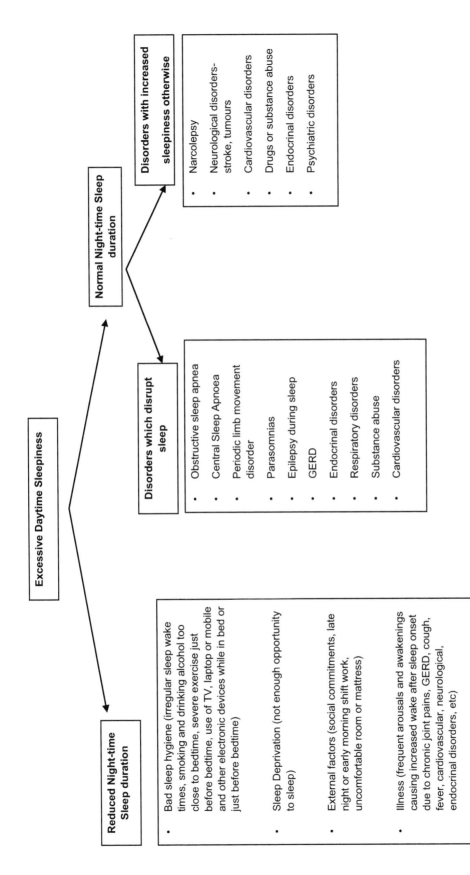

or sleep talking, kicks and jerks of the patient. Hence this history is sometimes as important as the history elicited from the patient. For example, the person may be only complaining of not feeling fresh after an adequate duration of sleep, but the bed partner mentions some abnormal movements in the patient's first one-third of night, thereby clinching the diagnosis of NREM parasomnias or giving a history of snoring and witnessed apnea indicating obstructive sleep apnea.

- **Associated daytime sleepiness and dysfunction:** Associated daytime consequences are frequently seen in sleep disorders due to reduced sleep duration or quality. Many disorders present with intense daytime sleepiness like sleep apnea, narcolepsy, sleep deprivation, etc. As discussed in the broad algorithm in the following figure, daytime sleepiness may be due to many causes related to sleep disorders or comorbidities causing sleep problems or even sleep disorders. The figure shows some of the important points to consider while working up a case of excessive daytime sleepiness.

  Excessive daytime sleepiness can be graded depending on the intensity with which it hampers daytime functioning and may vary from just feeling not fresh and looking for a reason to sleep to actually dozing off during an important task such as driving or working on machinery. The patient, due to lack of knowledge or awareness, may procrastinate the early reporting of daytime sleepiness and may end up in avoidable catastrophic accidents. Similarly, subtle decrements in daytime alertness or concentration and a dip in performance also follows a similar path if not enquired earlier in detail from the patient.

- **History of comorbidities:** Detailed history taking for clinical or subclinical presentations of various disorders that might impair sleep or cause disturbances in sleep may be required when the patient complaints are related to sleep. In clinical practice, before the disease presentation becomes evident, subtle symptoms and signs are often significant and lead to the early diagnosis and management of cases.

These are some of the important factors that must be kept in mind while approaching a case with sleep complaints. Apart from these broad factors, each patient may have personal predispositions and aggravating and relieving factors. It is always important to remember that an outpatient has an individualized set of problems and factors responsible for the symptoms that he is reporting. And sleep is a personal issue. Many factors play on one's mind, some more important than others, and hence a personalized evaluation will further help in the decision making and management of a patient's complaint of sleep problems.

CONCLUSION

This broad outline of common case presentations may be seen in outpatients and in wards while seeing patients with sleep complaints. A detailed workup is important to broadly categorize the type of sleep problem the patient is suffering from. This information is of extreme utility to the primary care physician in planning the course of management and referral of the patient if required.

SUGGESTED READING

1. American Academy of Sleep Medicine. *International Classification of Sleep Disorders*, 3rd ed. Darien, IL: American Academy of Sleep Medicine; 2014.

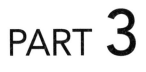

How Do I Investigate the Patient? (Assessment and Monitoring)

15

Basic Structure of Sleep Interview

DEEPAK SHRIVASTAVA, AND RICHA SHRIVASTAVA

THE STRUCTURED CLINICAL INTERVIEW

One of the most important components of patient evaluation with sleep complaints is the initial interview, which should be specific, goal directed, and comprehensive. A thorough sleep history outlining the nature of the complaint and screening for primary sleep disorders, as well as other medical and neurologic disorders, are crucial in creating the basic database that pervades the patient evaluation, clinical decision making, and establishing pretest probability and the appropriate selection of the diagnostic tests.

The *Structured Clinical Interview for Sleep Disorders (SCISD-R) for DSM-5 sleep disorders,* is a tool for the initial assessment of the most common sleep disorders. It was developed at the University of North Texas, USA. Although it has not been completely validated, it still provides a thorough framework that is designed to systematically document a patient's symptoms and the probability of the underlying disorders in an outpatient setting. This tool is easy for health practitioners to learn and use.

The clinical interview form includes multiple questions and takes about 10–20 minutes to administer. It covers nine major sleep disorders. Six of them have a high prevalence rate. The interrater reliability for these disorders, including insomnia, excessive sleepiness, obstructive sleep apnea, circadian rhythm sleep disorders, nightmares, and RLS disorder, is excellent.

The clinical interview is essential for the diagnosis of many sleep-wake disorders. In many of these disorders, the role of polysomnography is limited. A structured clinical interview is reliable and accurate to support the clinical decision making and proceed with evidence-based treatment selection.

DOI: 10.1201/9781003093381-18

While many structured or semi structured clinical interviews are available to assess sleep disorders, most of them have not been tested or validated.

While this instrument has many questions, any number of them can be skipped due to rule-outs. Eight questions related to typical sleep schedule are open ended. Subsequent questions assess every diagnostic symptom of the disorders previously mentioned and are rated:

Rating of 1: Absence of symptoms
Rating of 2: Possible presence of symptoms
Rating of 3: Definite presence of symptom
Rating of "?": Unsure

Interpretation: If necessary, DSM-5 symptoms are endorsed for a given diagnosis, and the patient is classified as having the disorder.

SLEEP INTERVIEW QUESTIONNAIRE

Date: _____
Referring Physician: _____ Last Name: _____ First Name: _____ Male/
Female _____ Marital Status: _____
M _____ S _____ W _____ D
Race _____ Date of birth: __/__/_____
Age: ___ Occupation_____
Emergency Contact and Phone

Section I: Main Complaint

1. What is your main sleep complaint?
2. How long has this been a problem?
3. Were there any events (weight gain, stress, illness, etc.) associated with the onset of your complaints?
4. Have you had a sleep study or home screen? ___ How long ago? ___ Where? _____
5. Have you ever used nasal CPAP or BiPAP? No ___ Yes ___ If so, how long? _____ Pressure setting _____ Mask _____

Section II: History of Sleep/Wake Disorder

General Sleep Wake assessment questions

Section III: Sleep Habits

1. What time do you go to bed on weekdays? _____ Weekends? _____

2. How long does it take you to fall asleep? _____
3. What percentage do you sleep on your Back ___% Stomach ___% Left/Right side ___/___%
4. a.) How often do you awaken at night? _____

   b.) How long do you stay awake? _____

   c.) What reason? (Bathroom, etc.) _____

5. What time do you get up on weekdays? _____ Weekends? _____
6. How many hours of sleep do you get in a typical night? _____
7. How do you feel in the morning?
   Very sleepy?   Sleepy, but   Wide awake
                  wake up soon   Ready to go
8. When do you function best?
   Morning: Best   Medium   Worst
   Afternoon: Best   Medium   Worst
   Evening: Best   Medium   Worst

Section IV: Medical History—Please outline your medical history:

Do you have or have ever been told you have:

- High Blood Pressure
- Elevated Cholesterol
- Migraine or Frequent Headaches
- Sinus Problems
- Stroke
- Parkinson's
- Diabetes
- GI Disease
- Dementia (Alzheimer's, etc.)
- Arthritis
- Cancer
- Prior History of Sleep Apnea
- Thyroid Problems
- Frequent Nighttime Urination
- Prior History of Restless Legs
- Anemia
- Depression and/or Anxiety
- Obesity
- Heart Disease
- Liver Disease
- Abnormal behavior during sleep
- Lung Disease
- Seizures or Epilepsy

Do you fall asleep or become sleepy when:	Never	Sometimes	Often	Always
1. Driving?	0	1	2	3
2 At work?	0	1	2	3
3 Do you take intentional naps?	0	1	2	3
4 Do you feel unable to move (paralyzed) when falling asleep?	0	1	2	3
5 Suddenly awaken choking for breath?	0	1	2	3
6 Grind your teeth?	0	1	2	3
7 Hold your breath? Or have you been told you stop breathing?	0	1	2	3
8 How would you rate your overall sleepiness?	0	1	2	3
9 Do you experience short periods of muscle weakness or loss of muscle control (especially with laughter or excitement)?	0	1	2	3
11 Do you think you need a sleeping pill, either prescription drug or over-the-counter sleeping aids in order to fall asleep?	0	1	2	3
11 Have nightmares?	0	1	2	3
12 Do you ever experience an uncomfortable or restless sensation in your legs when you relax or are first going to sleep that is relieved by moving or getting out of bed and walking?	0	1	2	3
13 Toss and turn or have restless sleep?	0	1	2	3
14 Walk or talk in your sleep? (Circle appropriate event.)	0	1	2	3
15 Snore?	0	1	2	3
16 Do you experience vivid dreamlike episodes when falling asleep?	0	1	2	3
17 Awaken with heartburn or acid reflux? (acid taste in mouth)	0	1	2	3
18 Wake up with a dry mouth?	0	1	2	3
19 Wake up with headaches?	0	1	2	3
20 Move about or engage in aggressive behaviors while asleep or awakening from sleep?	0	1	2	3
21 Do you consume wine or another alcoholic beverage in order to fall asleep?	0	1	2	3
22 Have you been taking sleeping pills or nonprescription sleeping aids on a nightly basis for more than three weeks?	0	1	2	3
23 Do you lay in bed for more than thirty minutes unable to go to sleep or return to sleep?	0	1	2	3
24 Do you dread getting into bed because you think you will "never" fall asleep?	0	1	2	3
25 How would you rate your overall sleepiness?	0	1	2	3

Past Medical or Surgical History (include all hospitalizations within the past five years)

Problem Date of onset Treatment Resolved/
                                    Current

_____

_____

_____

List prescription and over-the-counter medications/drugs patient is taking or recently has taken:

Name Dosage Frequency Reason

_____

_____

_____

_____

1. Patient weight? _____ Patient height? _____
2. Smoking Hx? _____ If yes, how long? _____ How much?___/ day
3. Alcohol use Hx? _____ If yes, how long? _____ How many drinks? ___/ day/wk/mo
4. Caffeinated beverage use (coffee, tea, soda)? _____ How many drinks? ___/ day/ wk/mo

General History

1. Reports of any other problems (e.g. stress, anxiety, or pressures)? If yes, explain:

_____

_____

2. Any changes in mood or irritability lately? If yes, explain:

_____

_____

3. Recent feelings of depression? If yes, explain:

_____

_____

4. Any recent problems with memory or concentration? If yes, explain:

_____

_____

5. Recent history of travel across time zones, that may affect sleep/wake schedule? If yes, explain:

_____

_____

6. Any sexual problems (impotency, lack of desire, premature ejaculation, etc.)? If yes, explain:

_____

_____

7. Any history of work night shifts and/or rotating shifts? If yes, explain:

_____

_____

HISTORY QUESTIONS DIVIDED INTO DIFFERENT CATEGORIES OF SLEEP DISORDERS

Screening Questions for Obstructive Sleep Apnea

- Snoring: Qualitative measures regarding loudness, changes in body position, factors exacerbating snoring and frequency
- Witnessed episodes of apnea: Frequency of the event, approximate length of the event, and observation of loud snoring or body jerks
- Awakening from the sleep with shortness of breath or a sense of choking
- Presence of night sweats
- Presence of morning headaches, frequency of headaches, and how long they last
- Number of nighttime awakenings: Most of the suspected causes of nighttime awakening and then inability to return to sleep
- Any changes in patient's weight, collar size, and presence of edema
- Severity of daytime sleepiness
- Circumstances and factors that worsen daytime sleepiness
- Number and the length of daytime naps
- Incidence of drowsy driving

This information can be substantiated with multiple screening tools that are available including the Epworth Sleepiness Scale, Stanford Sleepiness Scale, Visual Analog Scale, and STOP-BANG Questionnaire.

Screening Questions for Narcolepsy

Presence of excessive daytime sleepiness

Episodes of cataplexy manifested by muscle weakness, buckling of the knees, weakness in the arms, or jaw drop with intense emotional surge or excitement

Presence of hallucinations upon trying to fall asleep (In typical narcoleptic patients the sensations can be scary.)

Presence of sleep paralysis or inability to move while awakening from sleep

Presence of automatic behavior like driving a certain distance without the cognitive engagement or finding oneself at the place and not knowing how you get there

Screening Questions for Periodic Limb Movements of Sleep

Presence of leg cramps at bedtime

Experiencing crawling and an achy feeling in the legs during the latter part of the day or night with a feeling to get up and walk

Worsening of the leg discomfort during nighttime

Movement of the legs during the sleep observed by bed partner or others

Finding the bed covers in disarray

Sudden awakening with a jerk immediately after falling asleep

Screening Questions for Parasomnia

Recall of the dream of the event

Presence of nightmares

Episodes of acting out dreams with swinging arms, legs, moving, or yelling.

Approximate time of such activity during the night

Episodes of any injuries caused by these events and activity at night

History of sleepwalking

Approximate timing of sleepwalking during the night

History of sleep talking

Approximate timing of sleep talking during the night

Episodes of waking up from sleep in a state of confusion and disorientation

Screening Questions for Insomnia

Inability to fall asleep in 30 minutes or less after the lights are out

Episodes of waking up after falling asleep

Early morning awakening with shortening of the total sleep time

Inability to control racing thoughts and staying awake

Worry over time by watching the clock and inability to fall asleep

Any preoccupying thoughts causing anxiety and keeping wakefulness

Presence of chronic pain during the day or night

In addition, *International Classification of Sleep Disorders*, 3rd edition, further helps in providing guidelines for making the diagnosis of certain disorders. Once the diagnosis is suspected through the initial interview, the practitioner can follow the diagnostic criteria and get more information from the patient and the family.

Sleep Apnea Assessment Questionnaires

Sleep diary

Epworth Sleepiness Questionnaire

STOP-BANG Questionnaire

Berlin Questionnaire

Sleep Quality Assessment Questionnaires

Functional outcomes of sleep questionnaire (FOSQ)

Pittsburgh Sleep Quality Index (PHQ-9)

Restless Leg Syndrome Questionnaires

International Restless Legs Scale (IRLS)

Augmentation Severity Rating Scale (ASR S)

Restless Leg Syndrome Quality of Life Questionnaire (RLS Q OL)

Circadian Rhythm Questionnaires

Morningness-Eveningness Questionnaire (MEQ)

Munich Chronotype Questionnaire (MCT Q)

The Sleep Timing Questionnaire (ST Q)

Insomnia Assessment Questionnaires

Insomnia Severity Index (ISI)

Excessive Daytime Sleepiness Assessment

NARCOLEPSY

Stanford Sleepiness Scale (SSS)
Circle the ONE number that best describes your level of alertness or sleepiness RIGHT NOW.

1. Wide awake, fully awake, functioning at high level; head clear.
2. Functioning at a high level, but not at peak; able to concentrate.
3. Relaxed; awake; not at full alertness; responsive.
4. A little groggy; clearly not at peak; let down.
5. Fogginess; beginning to lose interest in remaining awake; slowed down.
6. Sleepiness; prefer to be lying down; fighting sleep, woozy.
7. Almost in reverie; sleep onset soon; lost struggle to remain awake.

CATAPLEXY QUESTIONNAIRE

This questionnaire determined that cataplexy was best differentiated from other types of muscle weakness when triggered by only three typical situations: "when hearing and telling a joke," "while laughing," or "when angry." The face or neck, rather than the limbs, were also more specifically involved in clear-cut cataplexy. This detailed questionnaire is available freely on the Internet.

ALLERGIES

Allergies have a significant impact on sleep and can worsen multiple sleep conditions. A detailed history of allergies is important, for both diagnostic and therapeutic purposes.

- Allergic rhinitis is a common complaint in approximately 40% of individuals.
- Insomnia is twice as likely in patients who have concomitant allergies.
- Nasal congestion, sneezing, and watery eyes tend to worsen at night and cause difficulty in breathing and poor-quality sleep.
- Interrupted sleep causes daytime tiredness and impairs performance.

- Allergies can cause insomnia, trouble falling asleep, and staying asleep.
- Allergies can cause increased snoring and a high risk of sleep apnea.
- Allergies lead to poor sleep efficiency and shortened total sleep time.

REVIEW OF SYSTEMS

Constitutional: Excessive daytime sleepiness tiredness and fatigue, no night sweats, no weight changes
Sleep: No insomnia, no early awakening, no interrupted sleep, refreshing normal sleep, no morning headaches
Eyes: No visual problems, no glaucoma, no eye pain
HENT: No deformities, no surgeries, no sneezing, congestion, runny nose, or sore throat, snoring.
Cardiovascular: No palpitations or edema
Respiratory: No shortness of breath, cough, wheezing
Gastrointestinal: No GERD, abdominal bloating, no nocturnal eating
Neurological: No morning headache, no sleep paralysis, no muscle weakness (cataplexy)
Musculoskeletal: No nighttime muscle activity/cramps, back pain, joint pain or stiffness
Hematologic: No anemia, bleeding, or bruising.
Lymphatic: No enlarged nodes
Endocrinologic: No reports of sweating, cold or heat intolerance, no polyuria or polydipsia
Psychiatric: No anxiety, no depression, no confusion or hallucinations
Skin: No rash, no masses
Allergies: No history of hives, eczema, or rhinitis

SLEEP HYGIENE

What time does the patient go to bed and what time does he or she usually awaken during the weekends, as well as on weekdays. See if the time remains constant or not.

NOCTURNAL AWAKENINGS

How many times does the patient wake up during sleep, and if so, what part of the night is it, and what are the usual causes—to urinate, shortness of breath, heartburn, body jerking, or not sure?

WORK SCHEDULE

Is the patient a shift worker?

Does he or she work swing shifts (shift changes from one week to the next)?

Recent travel history, especially resulting in jet lag and especially after traveling eastward

CIRCADIAN RHYTHM

Any trouble waking up in the morning?

Does the patient stay up later (i.e., 2–3 a.m.) and sleep in until noon? (*Delayed sleep phase—more common in adolescents*)

Does the patient go to bed at 8 p.m. and wake up at 3 a.m.? (*Advanced phase syndrome—more common in the elderly*)

FAMILY HISTORY

Family history is important as many disorders like narcolepsy run in families.

HABITS

Caffeine use in terms of quantity, frequency, and the time day

Alcohol use in terms of amount and relationship to bedtime

Smoking in terms of packs per day and for how many years

PHYSICAL EXAMINATION

A good-quality patient interview leads to a focused and specific examination of the patient, increasing the odds of capturing all the abnormalities. It also helps to design a proper diagnostic test that will support the initial diagnostic hypothesis.

In general, a sleep-related physical examination includes:

- Weight, height, and body mass index (BMI), and neck collar size (circumference) in centimeters.

- Head and neck exam of nasopharynx for nasopharyngeal edema, turbinate hypertrophy, or deviated nasal septum
- Examination of the teeth and dentition
- Anatomy of maxilla and mandible
- Retrognathia?
- Thick tongue?
- Anterior and posterior tonsillar pillars, soft palate, and uvula to assess for significant retropalatal obstruction with a narrow airway
- Systemic cardiac, pulmonary, and neurological examination

The review of sleep history and the interview of the patient and the assessment of the sleep complaint is one of the best tools available to establish a hypothesis and high pretest probability of the prospective diagnosis. It incorporates the predisposing and precipitating factors, other factors that exacerbate the symptoms, and the perceived impact of the symptoms on a patient's daytime functioning. As previously described, multiple diagnostic and screening instruments are available to assist in obtaining a reasonably reliable and comprehensive history.

SUGGESTED READING

1. Maurice M, Ohayon MD. Epidemiological overview of sleep disorders in the general population. *Sleep Med Res (SMR)*. 2011;2(1):1–9.
2. Dinges D. Recognizing problem sleepiness in your patients. *Am Fam Physician*. 1999;59(4):937–944.
3. Klingman KJ, Jungquist CR, Perlis ML. Questionnaires that screen for multiple sleep disorders. *Sleep Med Rev*. 2017;32:37–44. http://doi.org/10.1016/j.smrv.2016.02.004
4. El-Sayed IH. Comparison of four sleep questionnaires for screening obstructive sleep apnea. *Egypt J Chest Dis Tuberc*. 2012;61(4):433–441. https://doi.org/10.1016/j.ejcdt.2012.07.003.

Questionnaires

KARUNA DATTA

INTRODUCTION

In a clinical interview, after a detailed history taking and examination, the doctor often needs a tool to help in the diagnosis of the patient. Questionnaires thus are a necessary part of the armamentarium. Against the background of increased frequency of sleep-related complaints, they can be extremely useful.

TYPES OF QUESTIONNAIRES

Questionnaires can be broadly divided according to:

- Who completes them, i.e., whether they are:
  - Self-reported
  - Evaluated by a trained person
- The age of the patient, i.e., whether the patient is:
  - An infant
  - A child
  - An adolescent
  - An adult
- For what it is administered, e.g.:
  - Habits survey
  - Symptom questionnaire
- Disorder assessment questionnaire
- What it measures, e.g.:
  - Sleep quality
  - Assesses sleep apnea
  - Restless leg syndrome
  - Circadian rhythm
  - Insomnia
  - Daytime sleepiness

COMMON QUESTIONNAIRES USED IN CLINICAL PRACTICE

In the following paragraphs, we briefly discuss some commonly used questionnaires.

1. **Pittsburg Sleep Quality Index Questionnaire:** This questionnaire is filled out by the individual keeping in mind the past 1 month. It is meant for an adult to assess sleep quality. It has various subsections in which the subject mentions the usual sleep habits, the amount of trouble that few of the usual sleep problems, like coughing, bad dreams, inability to sleep, etc., cause on a scale of "not during the past month" to "three or more times a week." It has a question that subjectively marks the sleep quality of the patient. The patient is also asked to mark any history of medications taken for the problem or any symptoms like leg movements, snoring, etc. Overall, a global scale is given, by which >5 implies poor sleep quality. It is a sleep quality assessment tool [1].

2. **Epworth Sleepiness Scale:** This scale measures the chances of dozing off or falling asleep in 8 different situations or activities that most people engage in as part of their daily lives. It

DOI: 10.1201/9781003093381-19

is self-rated by the individual and measures sleepiness from the score calculated [2].

3. **Pre-Sleep Arousal Scale (PSAS):** This is a 16-item questionnaire that yields separate scale scores for physiological arousal and cognitive arousal. The PSAS is rated on a 5-point scale from 1 (not at all) to 5 (extremely), with items reflecting autonomic arousal on the PSAS physiological scale (e.g., heart racing/pounding, tight/tense muscles) and mental arousal on the PSAS cognitive scales (e.g., worry about not falling asleep, being mentally alert). It can be self-reported [3].

4. **Morningness Eveningness Scale (MES):** This instrument has 19 items. Questions are framed in a preferential manner, where respondents are asked to indicate when, for example, they would prefer to wake up or start sleep, rather than when they do. Depending on the scores calculated from the responses, it assesses morning or evening preferences [4].

5. **Depression Anxiety Stress Scale (DASS):** This instrument has 42 items and measures depression, anxiety, and stress over a period of 1 week. Each of the three DASS scales contains 14 items, divided into subscales of 2–5 items with similar content. Subjects are asked to use 4-point severity/frequency scales to rate the extent to which they have experienced each state over the past week. Scores for depression, anxiety, and stress are calculated by summing the scores for the relevant items [5].

6. **Insomnia Severity Index (ISI):** This instrument has seven items and is self-reported by patients. It is designed to assess the nature, severity, and impact of insomnia and monitor treatment response in adults over the past 2-week period [6, 7].

7. **Berlin Questionnaire [8] or the STOP-BANG Questionnaire [9]:** These can be used to assess sleep.

8. **Pictorial Sleepiness Scale Based on Cartoon Faces:** This self-reported questionnaire can be used for ages 4–73 years. It is an easy to administer instrument because it has cartoon faces showing the emotional state of the person reporting, and even with minimal literary skills, one can complete it [10].

9. **Children's Sleep Habits Questionnaire (CSHQ) [11], School Sleep Habits Survey (SSHS) [12], and Brief Infant Sleep Questionnaire (BISQ) [13]:** These are some of the common survey/habits questionnaires that can be used.

10. **Pediatric Sleep Questionnaire [14], Pediatric Daytime Sleepiness Scale [15], Stanford Sleepiness Scale [16], ESS [2], Cleveland Adolescent Sleepiness Questionnaire [17], and ESS for Children and Adolescents [18]:** These are some of the sleepiness evaluation scales.

11. **Morningness-Eveningness Questionnaire [4, 19], Munich Chronotype Questionnaire (MCTQ) [20], and The Sleep Timing Questionnaire (STQ) [21]:** These can be used to evaluate circadian rhythm.

12. **International Restless Leg Scale (IRLS):** This is a self-reported scale that has 10 questions and is developed to get a score based on assessment of the intensity and frequency of restless legs syndrome apart from its primary features and any other related problems. The score is obtained to scale the condition [22].

13. **Restless Legs Syndrome Quality of Life Questionnaire (RLSQoL):** This is another scale that can be used for assessing the disease [23].

14. **Tayside Children's Sleep Questionnaire:** This questionnaire was developed to assess sleep onset and sleep maintenance disorders in children of 1–5 years [24].

15. **Dysfunctional Beliefs and Attitudes Scale (DBAS):** These 16 items self-reported scale evaluates maladaptive cognitions that help perpetuate insomnia. It is a tool commonly used by cognitive behavioral therapists for treating insomnia [25].

Many other instruments are available. The things to keep in mind while picking an instrument for use are:

- The age group it is validated for.
- Condition or factors it is meant for.
- Permissions to use (contact person, whether free or restricted after obtaining permission).
- Ensuring the scores are calculated using the prescribed way in the validating study.

CONCLUSION

Questionnaires are an essential tool to evaluate sleep and sleep-related issues. The various factors to keep in mind while choosing the questionnaire are important.

REFERENCES

1. Buysse DJ, Reynolds CF, Monk TH, Berman SR, Kupfer DJ. The Pittsburgh sleep quality index: a new instrument for psychiatric practice and research. *Psychiatry Res.* 1989;28(2):193–213.

2. Johns MW. A new method for measuring daytime sleepiness: the Epworth sleepiness scale. *Sleep.* 1991;14(6):540–545.

3. Nicassio PM, Mendlowitz DR, Fussell JJ, Petras L. The phenomenology of the pre-sleep state: the development of the pre-sleep arousal scale. *Behav Res Ther.* 1985;23(3):263–271.

4. Horne JA, Ostberg O. A self-assessment questionnaire to determine Morningness-Eveningness in human circadian rhythms. *Int J Chronobiol.* 1976;4(2):97–110.

5. Lovibond PF, Lovibond SH. The structure of negative emotional states: comparison of the Depression Anxiety Stress Scales (DASS) with the Beck Depression and Anxiety Inventories. *Behav Res Ther.* 1995;33(3):335–343.

6. Morin CM, Belleville G, Bélanger L, Ivers H. The Insomnia Severity Index: psychometric indicators to detect insomnia cases and evaluate treatment response. *Sleep.* 2011;34(5):601–608.

7. Bastien CH, Vallières A, Morin CM. Validation of the insomnia severity index as an outcome measure for insomnia research. *Sleep Med.* 2001;2(4):297–307.

8. Netzer NC, Stoohs RA, Netzer CM, Clark K, Strohl KP. Using the Berlin Questionnaire to identify patients at risk for the sleep apnea syndrome. *Ann Intern Med.* 1999;131(7):485.

9. Chung F, Yegneswaran B, Liao P, Chung SA, Vairavanathan S, Islam S, et al. STOP questionnaire. *Anesthesiology.* 2008;108(5):812–821.

10. Maldonado CC, Bentley AJ, Mitchell D. A pictorial sleepiness scale based on cartoon faces. *Sleep.* 2004;27(3):541–548.

11. Owens JA, Spirito A, McGuinn M. The Children's Sleep Habits Questionnaire (CSHQ): psychometric properties of a survey instrument for school-aged children. *Sleep.* 2000;23(8):1043–1051.

12. Wolfson AR, Carskadon MA. Sleep schedules and daytime functioning in adolescents. *Child Dev.* 1998;69(4):875–887.

13. Sadeh A. A brief screening questionnaire for infant sleep problems: validation and findings for an internet sample. *Pediatrics.* 2004;113(6):e570–e577.

14. Chervin RD, Hedger K, Dillon JE, Pituch KJ. Pediatric sleep questionnaire (PSQ): validity and reliability of scales for sleep-disordered breathing, snoring, sleepiness, and behavioral problems. *Sleep Med.* 2000;1(1):21–32.

15. Drake C, Nickel C, Burduvali E, Roth T, Jefferson C, Pietro B. The pediatric daytime sleepiness scale (PDSS): sleep habits and school outcomes in middle-school children. *Sleep.* 2003;26(4):455–458.

16. Hoddes E, Zarcone V, Smythe H, Phillips R, Dement WC. Quantification of sleepiness: a new approach. *Psychophysiology.* 1973;10(4):431–436.

17. Spilsbury JC, Drotar D, Rosen CL, Redline S. The Cleveland adolescent sleepiness questionnaire: a new measure to assess excessive daytime sleepiness in adolescents. *J Clin Sleep Med.* 2007;3(6):603–612.

18. Janssen KC, Phillipson S, O'Connor J, Johns MW. Validation of the Epworth Sleepiness Scale for children and adolescents using Rasch analysis. *Sleep Med.* 2017;33:30–35.

19. Paine SJ, Gander PH, Travier N. The epidemiology of morningness/eveningness: influence of age, gender, ethnicity, and socioeconomic factors in adults (30–49 years). *J Biol Rhythms.* 2006;21(1):68–76.

20. Roenneberg T, Wirz-Justice A, Merrow M. Life between clocks: daily temporal patterns of human chronotypes. *J Biol Rhythms.* 2003;18(1):80–90.

21. Monk TH, Buysse DJ, Kennedy KS, Potts JM, DeGrazia JM, Miewald JM. Measuring sleep habits without using a diary: the sleep timing questionnaire. *Sleep.* 2003;26(2):208–12.

22. Walters AS, LeBrocq C, Dhar A, Hening W, Rosen R, Allen RP, Trenkwalder C. Validation of the international restless legs syndrome study group rating scale for restless legs syndrome. *Sleep Med.* 2003;4(2):121–132.

23. Abetz L, Vallow SM, Kirsch J, Allen RP, Washburn T, Earley CJ. Validation of the restless legs syndrome quality of life questionnaire. *Value Health.* 2005;8(2):157–167.

24. McGreavey JA, Donnan PT, Pagliari HC, Sullivan FM. The Tayside children's sleep

questionnaire: a simple tool to evaluate sleep problems in young children. *Child Care Health Dev.* 2005;31(5):539–544.

25. Morin CM, Vallières A, Ivers H. Dysfunctional beliefs and attitudes about sleep (DBAS): validation of a brief version (DBAS-16). *Sleep.* 2007;30(11):1547–1554.

SUGGESTED READING

1. Shahid A, Wilkinson K, Marcu S, Shapiro CM, editors. *STOP, THAT and One Hundred Other Sleep Scales.* New York and Heidelberg: Springer; 2014. 421 p.

Use of a Sleep Diary

KARUNA DATTA

INTRODUCTION

A sleep diary is an important instrument to log both daytime activities and sleep over a period. Preferably the sleep diary should be maintained for 14 days. In follow-up cases, it may be done for 7 days. The most important aspect of a complete sleep diary is the motivated person who creates it. The primary care physician or the therapist needs to spend time making the patient understand the need to fill out the diary regularly to get a complete diary, and if the patient does miss a day for some unavoidable reason, a page may be left blank rather than trying to complete it by retrospective recall. A sleep diary requires prospective recall, and hence it should be filled twice daily, once just before the sleep time when the patient writes about the daytime activities and then immediately after waking up when the patient gives details about the nighttime sleep pattern. The sleep diary is recommended to be used throughout an intervention or a therapy session to understand the change in habits and in sleep-wake and thus to study the effect of intervention. This chapter discusses the methodology of using a sleep diary and the sleep diary of a case of chronic insomnia.

WHAT IS A SLEEP DIARY?

A sleep diary is a methodical log of sleep and wake-related activities, habits, and feelings over the entire 24-hour period. Ideally, it should be filled out for 14 days.

LOGGING THE SLEEP DIARY

Methodology

The adult can complete his or her own diary. In case of a child, the caregiver can fill in the details. Essentially, the entry in the sleep diary should be done as immediately as possible to avoid a recall issue. Prospective sleep diaries are better than retrospective diaries, and hence this logging should be done immediately. The diary should include details about the activities during daytime, for example, exercise, food habits, general feelings of the day, nap details, coffee intake, etc. Any other significant history like that of smoking, alcohol intake should also be included with details. These daytime activities should be recorded just before going to sleep. The details about the sleep and the

DOI: 10.1201/9781003093381-20

routine followed should be entered immediately after getting up in the morning. Sleep is considered to change, and no one night is the same. Hence filling in the details about sleep should be completed by the patient immediately after getting up. Also, it must be emphasized to the patient that the sleep diary should be written twice in a 24-hour period, i.e., about the wake activities just before going off to sleep and about sleep time just after waking up.

Types of Diaries

The sleep diary can be a pictographic representation where one can mark awake with standing arrow and lying in bed to sleep as an inverted arrow. The sleep period can be shaded and awake kept unshaded. One can write on timeline the different activities one performed like exercise, mealtime, etc. An AASM 2-week diary is available to use freely.

A second type may be again a paper type but descriptive, wherein the patient describes daytime activities and sleep time. Space is provided where the patient writes in descriptive detail. Though it is time-consuming to both enter and analyze, it has an advantage of revealing many other fine details that the patient might like to share or be told to elaborate on.

The third may be an e-type of either of the preceding two types, with provision for marking as pictogram on an interactive PDF, Word document, etc., or an Excel sheet where the same space can be used to describe the events in detail.

Instructions to Patient about Logging

A sleep diary, if filled in correctly by the patient, is a valuable tool in the assessment and evaluation of sleep disorders and its treatment. It is inexpensive and easy to do. The effectiveness of this method lies in the hands of the patient who is filling in the details. At times, just handing over the sleep diary confuses the patient unless properly explained. Next, some basic concepts are explained regarding the need for completion, as these points must be elaborated on for the patient to be motivated to complete the diary.

The need to make entries regularly, twice a day, and for a minimum of 14 days is to be emphasized to the patient. There are two broad blocks: wake activities and sleep time patterns.

Wake Activities in the Sleep Diary

The patient should write just before going to sleep. The first to note down is about exercise during wake time. The severity of exercise can affect sleep; for example, if exercise is very severe, it affects sleep differently than mild or moderate exercise. The duration of exercise is also important. Another factor that plays an important role as far as exercise is concerned is the time of the day it is being done. Exercising too close to bedtime may be a problem in sleep initiation for some patients. Scientific literature shows ambiguous results and high-intensity exercises have been found to cause initiation in sleep problems in some and improvement in sleep in some studies of OSA patients. Though mild to moderate exercise is known to help sleep. Also, an exercise routine in the morning may help in advancing sleep at night and may delay sleep for some when done in the evening. A factor that plays an important role is the patient's chronotype. As previously discussed about sleep consultations in Chapter 15, questions for chronotype preference may be used to help understand the influence of chronotype, the type of exercise, and the timing of exercise on sleep.

Night sleep may be affected by nap durations during the day. It is vital to motivate the patient to note the duration and the time of the nap. Nap time may be a significant factor itself during therapy. A chronic insomnia patient who is unable to sleep at night may take a nap in the afternoon for a few hours, which may affect his sleep at night and hence cause a vicious cycle of bad sleep, leading to increased nap times and further worsening of sleep.

The number of cups of tea and coffee is important to document. The patient may be asked to note the timing of the last cup of tea or coffee. This may be important to notice since a delayed time of tea or coffee might be the cause of affecting sleep. Similarly, alcohol intake needs to be documented. Alcohol is often considered by the patient as a mechanism to smooth over problems of the day or sometimes is even used to aid sleep. This misconception must be clarified to the patient, who should be told clearly that alcohol actually affects sleep by deteriorating the maintenance of sleep at night. Therefore, documentation of alcohol consumption helps the caregiver to compare the night sleep based on the days alcohol was consumed as compared to other days of the patient's diary.

The composition of meals and their timing play an important role. Foods rich in tryptophan and carbohydrates are known to enhance sleep. Take careful note of patients on dieting or weight loss plans. Acute alterations in food and water intake might be an important finding affecting sleep. Heavy meals just before sleep are known to hamper it. In cases of gastroesophageal reflux disease (GERD), recurrent arousals due to acid reflux might be seen, and these would be found to increase with meals very close to bedtime. Generally, meals should be lighter at night. Not so light as to cause awakening at night due to hunger and not so heavy that it causes discomfort and problems sleeping. Physiologically, food should be in the late digestion phase so that during sleep, insulin is starting to decline, and, when slow wave sleep sets in, the release of growth hormone causes repair. An ideal balance on the composition of meals and its timing is important in sleeping better, and hence logging it carefully in the diary is crucial.

Documenting feelings during the day is important because sleep can be affected by the feelings or mood of the person in the course of the day. Likewise, sleep can also affect the mood of the person. This bidirectional link is documented in literature and hence is important to study in the patient. Days when the patient is sad or tired as compared to feeling active may hold a clue about the effect of mood or feelings on sleep and vice versa.

It is also useful at times to complete this documentation by asking the patients to mention their mood just before sleep. Sometimes the day was active, but just before sleep the patient was tired; it may be important to note the sleep that day. It may be different compared to when the patient is sad the entire day but is calm just before going to sleep.

Medications that are taken regularly should be documented. Nonpharmacological sleep aids, e.g., warm milk, eye covers, etc. and pharmacological aids in the form of sedatives, hypnotics, or sleep-inducing or affecting drug should be mentioned. Cough syrups or antiallergic medications that are often taken by the patient sometimes are not documented, and that makes it very difficult to understand the varying pattern of sleep due to these commonly taken drugs. A detailed initial history should be taken, and the patient should be

educated about the importance of writing details of these aids in the sleep diary so that these important inputs are not missed.

Logging Sleep Time in the Sleep Diary

Just before going to sleep, the bedtime routine may be documented in the sleep diary. Bedtime is when the patient decides to go off to bed. For example, if the patient works from 10 p.m. to 11 p.m. in bed, at 11 p.m. switches off the light to go to sleep, and is asleep in approximately 5–10 minutes, then 11 p.m. is the bedtime, and the working from 10 p.m. to 11 p.m. is the bedtime routine, where it can be mentioned as "working on laptop from 10 p.m to 11 p.m." On the other hand, if the patient lies in the bed to sleep at 10 p.m., and is unable to sleep till 11 p.m., so gets up and works till 11:30, and then lies back down to sleep at 11:30 p.m., then bedtime is 10 p.m. The time from 10 p.m. to when he sleeps is the time he could not sleep. In this case the person can be told to write details of working from 11 to 11:30 p.m. in the column of time of "time in bed not able to sleep." Unless these details are elaborated by the patient, the treating health care provider does not come to know about these habits. Refer to sleep hygiene habits in Chapter 22. These habits need to be addressed. When this fact is realized by the patient also, it is easier for the patient to understand how to deal with it.

From bedtime onward, the patient is now instructed not to look at the watch for recording time but is instructed only to fill in the sleep diary in the morning, immediately after waking up.

Upon waking up, the patient fills in the diary the second time right away, this time about the sleep at night. The patient is supposed to write about bedtime, as discussed, then about wake-up time, that is, when he or she finally woke up and got out of bed. Time spent in bed not able to sleep is the approximate time after bedtime that one takes to get to sleep. So, in our first patient, the time spent in bed not sleeping, also called sleep onset latency, is 5–10 minutes, while in the second case, it is almost 1.5 hours from 10 p.m. to 11:30 p.m.

After this, one notes the number and duration of sleep breaks. The breaks in sleep that happens up to the time one finally wakes up are the sleep breaks. These are also called wake after sleep onset (WASO). These sleep breaks may be many but of small duration, or they may be only one or two but of long duration. The patient is instructed not to look at the watch at night but approximately mention the number of times he or she woke up during sleep and the duration of each break. The patient may also write down the approximate time of the night when the break probably happened. It is important to emphasize to the patient *not* to look at a watch or an alarm clock but rather to include all the details of the timing and duration of sleep breaks only by estimation.

After writing about the sleep breaks, the patient should mention the wake-up time, which is the time when she or he finally wakes up from the bed. This is the only time other than the bedtime when the patient is allowed to look at the watch.

WHAT CAN BE ASSESSED AND EVALUATED WITH A SLEEP DIARY

A well written sleep diary can help identify sleep problems and disorders like insomnia, sleep deprivation, and circadian rhythm disorders like delayed sleep-wake phase disorder, advanced sleep-wake phase disorder, shift work, etc., cases of hypersomnolence, conditions where sleep quality is reduced or abnormal occurrences, history of nightmares, etc.

CASE DISCUSSION

The Sleep Diary of a Chronic Insomnia Patient

A 62-year-old, doctor, with hypertension and diabetes already on medications, presented with complaints of inability to sleep after lying down to sleep in bed and intermittent waking up almost every night and then not being able to go back to sleep after that break or unable to sleep for long periods after waking up at night. He was on antihypertensives and antidiabetics regularly.

The patient has this history of almost 11 years. Detailed interview findings are not discussed here. The presentation is kept relevant to the sleep diary. However, to have a better understanding of the management of this case, it is suggested to read Chapters 6, 22, and 23. Figures 17.1–17.14 present the pages of the sleep diary kept during the course of treatment. The text that follows comments on the diary entries.

Timeline-wise Sleep Diary Details

- 14 Jan 2021–26 Jan 2021: Figures 17.1–17.4 show 2 weeks of a baseline sleep diary of daytime and sleep time data. A general history taking and physical examination were conducted. Notice that the patient exercised regularly, took a nap around 3–4 p.m. for almost an hour; sleep onset latency was more than 30 minutes for most nights. Wake after sleep onset, i.e., the amount of time the subject felt awake after falling off to sleep and finally waking up in the morning was also more than 30 minutes for most nights, and on some nights he could not sleep at all after waking up very early in the morning. His blood pressure was controlled by antihypertensives.

- 01 Feb 2021: The patient was told about the principles of sleep hygiene. His predisposing, perpetuating, and precipitating factors were explored during the interview by the physician, and a detailed case history regarding insomnia was taken. The patient used to measure his BP daily at home and thus was asked to mention it in the sleep diary. Stimulus control was explained, and the patient asked to follow it. He was asked to keep his nap earlier than 2:30 p.m.

- 08 Feb 2021: Yoga nidra intervention started for patient. The subjective effectiveness of yoga nidra session was asked to be documented to notice the effectiveness of the practice sessions. The diary as depicted in Figures 17.5 and 17.6 shows that naps had reverted back to the afternoon. Though sleep onset latency was better, WASO was still more than 30 minutes for most nights. Although the sleep quality mentioned was OK, on a rating scale it ranged from only 3 to 4.5 out of 10! Yoga nidra session effectiveness was only 30–35%, and this is where the supervised sessions and individualized approach was important to make them more effective. Details of the yoga nidra therapeutic model are available in further reading.

- 22 Feb 2021: The patient was taught how to do progressive muscular relaxation.

- 22 Mar–04 Apr 2021: Increased naps are seen in the diary (Figures 17.7–17.10). The patient felt excessively sleepy until 28 Mar. The patient reported that he did not have much improvement. However, some effect was visible

Sr. No.	Day (Pl add Date)	Monday 18/1/21	Tuesday 19/1/21	Wednesday 20/1/21	Thursday 14/1	Friday 15/1	Saturday 16/1	Sunday 17/1
1	Exercise (type and duration)	18/1/21 Nil	one hour wak in morning 10 min evening	one hr walk	one hr walk	Walk 50 min Stretching 10 min	No walk (Break)	walk for 35 min Stretching exercise
2	Naps (time and duration)	30 min 4PM to 4.30 PM	25 min in afternoon (1.30pm)	45 min 3pm - 3.45 pm	1500h - 1600 h for 20 min	-	30 min at - 4pm	35 min nap at 3.30pm
3	Alcohol (number of pegs)	-	-		-	-	one glass beer	-
4	Tea & Coffe (number of cups & last)	2 cups last at 5pm	-	2 1/2 cups	1 cup In evening	Total 2 cups Last - at 6 pm	02 cup (Last - cup at 5pm)	Total 2 cups Last - cup at 5 pm
5	Feelings	Better	Not great	Better	fell better in evening after naps	Not great	Better (In morning and afternoon)	ok
6	Food & Drink (time of meals)	Lunch - 2 PM Dinner - 8 PM	Lunch - 2 PM Dinner 9 PM	Lunch - 1PM Dinner - 8 PM	2 chapat, dal, curd 2 glass water Lunch-2PM Dinner- 8PM	Dinner at 8.30 PM	Lunch 2.30pm Dinner 8.15 PM	Lunch 1.30 p m Dinner 8 pm
7	Medications or sleep Aids	Hypertension Diabetes	Hypertension Diabetes	Hypertension Diabetes	Hypertension Diabetes	Hypertension diabetes	Hypertension Diabetes	Hypertension Diabetes
8	Bedtime Routine	TV 8pm - 9pm	TV 9.15 pm - 10pm	TV 7.30 pm - 8.30 pm	TV off - at 5pm no mobile 8pm 9pm	TV at 7pm - 8 pm no mobile Read a bed	No TV in evening	No TV

		Tuesday 19/1/21	Wednesday 20/1/21	Thursday 14/1	Friday 15/1	Saturday 16/1	Sunday 17/1	Monday 18/1
9	Bed Time	10.15 pm	10.30pm	9.30pm	9.30 pm	9.30 pm	9.45 pm	9.40. pm
10	Wake -up Time	0500h	0500h	0500h	0500h	4.30 Am	0500h	0.500h
11	Time spent in Bed initially trying to sleep after lying down	30 min	15 min	1 hr 15 min	50 min	50 min	30 min	25 min
12	Sleep Breaks number (duration)	one at 2.30 Am 45-50 min	one at 4 AM 30 min againslept for 25 min	Two (5 min) midnight 2.30 am (2 hrs)	one (20 min) 3.30 Am Got up at 4.30 Am	one at 1.30 am then Couldn't sleep	one at 2am then 35 min Got up at 5am	one at 2am then couldn't sleep
13	Quality of Sleep & Other Comments	Better	Good	poor Couldn't sleep after 2.30PM	Average	poor	Average	poor
14	Overall rating your sleep out of 10 (if 0 is no sleep and 10 is life best sleep)	5	5	3	4	3	4	3
15	Total sleep Hours	5 hrs 15 min	6 hrs approx 9.30PM	3 hrs	5 hr. 20 min	3 hrs	4 1/2 hrs	
			142/88	B.P 149/94 (9.30 pm) 152/90	B.P 152/92 (0500h)	5.30 am 155/44 9.15 pm 141/91	0500h 134/91 141/92	5 am 135/92 9.30 pm

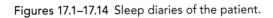

Figures 17.1–17.14 Sleep diaries of the patient.

Sr. No.	Day (Pl add Date)	Monday 25/11/21	Tuesday 26/11/21	Wednesday 27/1	Thursday 21/11/21	Friday 02/11/21	Saturday 23/1	Sunday 24/1
1	Exercise (type and duration)	Walk 1hr	one hr walk		one hr walk + 15min Stretching	1 hr walk	-	-
2	Naps (time and duration)	50min at 4pm	40 min 3pm		20 min at 3.30 pm	-	2 hr 2pm-4pm	1pm-2pm 1hr
3	Alcohol (number of pegs)	-	—		Nil	Nil	one glass Beer	-
4	Tea & Coffe (number of cups & last	2½ cups	2½ cups		1½ morning 1 cup evening	2½ cups (morning & evening)	2½ cups Total	2 cups morning 1 cup evening
5	Feelings	Good	ok		Good	ok	Better	Better
6	Food & Drink (time of meals)	lunch 1300h dinner at 8.30 pm	lunch 2.30pm Dinner 8.30pm		lunch 2pm Dinner 8 pm	lunch 1pm Dinner a pm	lunch 1.30pm Dinner a pm	lunch 2pm Dinner 9pm
7	Medications or sleep Aids	Hypertension Diabetes	Hypertension Diabetes		Hypertension Diabetes	Hypertension Diabetes	Hypertension Diabetes	Hypertension Diabetes
8	Bedtime Routine	TV 8pm ↓	TV 8.30pm		TV 7.30pm ↓	TV 8pm ↓	No TV	TV 7pm
		5:15 Am 143/94 9.15 pm 141/90	5 Am 136/94 9.30 pm 156/96		5 Am 141/94 10pm 143/94	5 Am 149/90	5 Am 143/95 9.45 pm 148/92	05 Am 129/92 158/96

		Tuesday 26/11/21	Wednesday 27/11/21	Thursday 21/1/21	Friday 22/1	Saturday 23/1	Sunday 24/1/21	Monday 25/11/21
9	Bed Time	10 pm		9.45 pm	9→ 10pm	10.30 pm	10.30 pm	10pm.
10	Wake-up Time	0500h		0500h	5.15 am	5.00 am	5.15 am	4 am
11	Time spent in Bed initially trying to sleep after lying down	2 hrs		20min	45 min	20 min	1 hr	20min
12	Sleep Breaks number (duration)	Two 2am(30min) 3.30am didn't sleep after 3.30am		one at 3.45 am	one at 2 am 1hr-30 min	Two 2.30am hr 4.30am	Two 2.30 AM 45 min 4.30AM	one at 4am slept at 4.30 For ½ h.
13	Quality of Sleep & Other Comments	poor		Good (best in last 9 days)	not great	ok	ok	good
14	Overall rating your sleep out of 10 (if 0 is no sleep and 10 is life best sleep)	3		5	3	4	4	5
15	Total sleep Hours	approx 4 hrs		6 hours	4hrs 45min	5hrs 30 min	5hr	6hrs 45min
								5 am 13c/94

Figures 17.1–17.14 (Continued)

Yoga Nidra Started

Sr. No.	Day (Pl add Date)	Monday 8|2	Tuesday 9|2	Wednesday 10|2	Thursday 11|2	Friday 5|2|21	Saturday 6|2	Sunday 7|2
1	Exercise (type and duration)	1 hr	—	—	walk 40 min	walk 1 hour	—	—
2	Naps (time and duration)	1 hour 2.30-3pm 30 min	1 hour 3-4 pm	1 hour 2-3 pm	30 min 4-4.30pm	1 hr 2pm -3pm	1 hr 2-3pm	45 min 2-2.45 pm
3	Alcohol (number of pegs)	—	—	—	—	—	one glass beer	—
4	Tea & Coffe (number of cups & last	2 1/2 cups last cd 5pm	2 cups last cd 4.30pm	2 cups last cd 4.30pm	2 cups	2 1/2 cups	2 1/2 cups	2 1/2 cups
5	Feelings	ok	ok	ok	ok	ok	Not good	ok
6	Food & Drink (time of meals)	lunch - 1pm Dinner- 8.40pm	lunch - 1pm Dinner - 7.45pm	lunch - 1pm Dinner- 8.30pm	lunch 1pm Dinner 8pm	lunch 12.45pm Dinner 8pm	lunch 1pm Dinner 8.45pm	lunch 1pm Dinner 8.15pm
7	Medications or sleep Aids	Hypertensi-on Diabetes	Hypertension Diabetes	Hypertension Diabetes	Hypertension Diabetes	Hypertension Diabetes	Hypertension Diabetes	Hypertension Diabetes
8	Bedtime Routine	TV 7.30pm One hour	TV 9 pm (one hour)	TV 8pm (one hour)	TV 9pm (one hour)	TV 8 pm (one hour)	No TV	TV 8.30pm (1 hour)

5.00 AM	5.30am	5.30 am	5.30am	5.30 AM	5.30 AM	5.30 AM
138|84	146|93	141|94	135|90	137|84	141|92	140|9|
9pm .147|94	9pm 146|89	9.30pm 139|87	9.30pm 156|93	9.30 pm 140|96	9.30 pm 148|87	

		Tuesday 9|2	Wednesday 10|2	Thursday 11|5	Friday 5|2|21	Saturday 6|2|21	Sunday 7|2	Monday 8|2
9	Bed Time	9.30 pm	9.40 pm	10.15 pm	10 pm	10 pm	9.45 pm	9.30 pm
10	Wake -up Time	5.30 am	5.30 am	5 am	5.00 am	5.30 am	5.25 am	4.30 am
11	Time spent in Bed initially trying to sleep after lying down	15 min	20 min	20 min	20 min	20 min	20 min approx	1 hour
12	Sleep Breaks number (duration)	one 3am for 1hr slept for 30 min against	one 3 am for 1hr slept again for 45min	Two 1.30am 30 min 3.30am	one 3.30am 20 min approx	one 1.30am then did'nt sleep	one at 4 am 20 min	one at 1.30 am then did'nt sleep
13	Quality of Sleep & Other Comments	ok	ok	poor	ok	poor	ok	poor
14	Overall rating your sleep out of 10 (If 0 is no sleep and 10 is life best sleep)	4-5	4.5	3	4	3	4.5	3
15	Total sleep Hours	5 1/2 hr	6hr 45min	4 1/2 hrs	6hrs 45 min	3 1/2 hrs	approx 7 hrs	3hr

yoga nidra 30\|100

yoga nidra 35\|100

Figures 17.1–17.14 (Continued)

Sr. No.	Day (Pl add Date)	Monday 22/3	Tuesday 23/3	Wednesday 24/3	Thursday 25/3	Friday 26/3	Saturday 27/3	Sunday 28/3
1	Exercise (type and duration)	1 hr	–	–	–	1 hr	–	1+1½ hr
2	Naps (time and duration)	1+½ hr 12-1·30pm	1+½ hr 9-10·30 Am	1 hr 2-3 pm	2 hrs 10-12 Am	1+½ hr 12-1·30pm	2h 11-1 pm	1+1½ hr 2·30-4pm
3	Alcohol (number of pegs)	–	–	–	–	–	Beer one glass	–
4	Tea & Coffe (number of cups & last)	3 cups last at 6pm	3 cups last at 5PM	2 ½ cups last at 6PM	2 cups last at 6·30 pm	3 cups last at 2pm	2 ½ cups last at	3 cups last at 6 pm
5	Feelings	OK	ok	ok	Better	OK	ok	Better
6	Food & Drink (time of meals)	lunch - 2pm Dinner 8·30pm	lunch- 2pm Dinner 8pm	lunch 1·30pm Dinner 7·45pm	lunch – 1·30pm Dinner- 8pm	lunch – 2pm Dinner 8·15pm	lunch - 2pm Dinner 9pm	lunch - 1·30pm Dinner 8·45pm
7	Medications or sleep Aids	Hypertension Diabetes	Hypertension Diabetes	Hypertensi on Diabetes	Hypertension Diabetes	Hypertensi on Diabetes	Hypertensi on Diabetes	Hypotensi on Diabetes
8	Bedtime Routine	TV 9pm (1 hour)	TV 8pm (1 hours)	TV 8 pm (1 hour)	TV 8pm (1 hour)	TV 8pm (1 hour)	TV 10pm (1 hour)	TV 10·30pm (1 hour)

5·30 Am
BP 127/78
Yoga nidna
Tr 100
pm. 131/82

5·30 Am
129/86
Yoga nidna
70/100
9pm 126/82

129/80
yoga nidna
65/100
9·30pm132/82

5 am
126/86
yoga nidna
69/100

126/82
5·30am
Yoga nidna
65/100
9·15 Pm 132/86

135/84
yoga nidna
60/100

129/86
yoga nidna
60/100
132/81

		Tuesday 23/3	Wednesday 24/3	Thursday 25/3	Friday 26/3	Saturday 27/3	Sunday 28/3	Monday 22/3
9	Bed Time	10pm	10pm	11pm	10·30 pm	11 pm	11 pm	10·30 pm
10	Wake -up Time	5 am	5 am	4 am	5 am	4·15 am	4·15 am	5 am
11	Time spent in Bed initially trying to sleep after lying down	15 min	20 min	15 min	30 min	10 min	10 min	30 min
12	Sleep Breaks number (duration)	one at 4 am 1 hr	one at 3·50am 30 min	one at 4 am (Got up at 6am)	Two 2 am 1 hr 4·15am	–	–	one 2·15 am 45 min slept ag-ain
13	Quality of Sleep & Other Comments	Better	Better	Better	Bad	Better	Better	ok
14	Overall rating your sleep out of 10 (if 0 is no sleep and 10 is life best sleep)	4·5	4·5	4·5	3·5	4·5	5	4
15	Total sleep Hours	5hrs 45 min	6 ½ hr	6hr 45 min	5 hrs	5 ½ hr	6 hrs	6 hrs

Figures 17.1–17.14 (Continued)

Sr. No.	Day (Pl add Date)	Monday 29.3	Tuesday 30.3	Wednesday 31.3	Thursday 1.4	Friday 2.4	Saturday 3.4	Sunday 4.4
1	Exercise (type and duration)	1 hr	1½ hr	1 hr 20 min	1 hr	1 hr	–	½ hr
2	Naps (time and duration)	1 hr 12-1 pm	1½ hr 11-12.30 pm	30 min 2-2.30 pm	1 hr 2-3 pm	2 hr 11-1 pm	45 min 1-1.45 pm	1½ hr 11.30-1 pm
3	Alcohol (number of pegs)	–	–	–	–	–	–	–
4	Tea & Coffe (number of cups & last	3 cups 5.30 pm	2 cups 4.30 pm	3 cups 5.30 pm	3 cups 6 pm	2 cups	2 cups 4 pm	3 cups
5	Feelings	OK	ok	OK	ok	ok	ok	OK
6	Food & Drink (time of meals)	lunch - 2 pm Dinner 8.30 pm	lunch - 2 pm Dinner 8 pm	lunch 1.45 pm Dinner 9 pm	lunch 12.45 pm Dinner 8 pm	lunch 2 pm Dinner 7.30 pm	lunch 2 pm Dinner 8 pm	lunch 1.30 pm Dinner 8 pm
7	Medications or sleep Aids	Hypertension Diabetes	Hypertension Diabetes	Hypertension Diabetes	Hypertension Diabetes	Hypertension Diabetes	Hypertension Diabetes	Hypertension Diabetes
8	Bedtime Routine	TV 8.30 pm (one hour)	TV 9 pm (one hour)	TV 8.30 pm (one hour)	TV 7.30 pm (one hour)	TV 8 pm (one hour)	TV 9 pm (one hour)	TV 9.30 pm (one hour)

8.30
128/82
yoga nidra
60 |100
9 pm
131 179

5 Am
135 |90
yoga
Nidra
65 |100
9.30 131/85

129/86

130/85
yoga 70/
Nidna
128/78
10 pm

5.30
134/82
yoga nidna
80 |100
9.45 123/82

5.00
135/85
10 pm
126/82

5.30
132/85
yoga nidna
70 |100
10.30 pm
128/87

		Tuesday 30.3	Wednesday 31.3	Thursday 1.4	Friday 2.4	Saturday 3.4	Sunday 4.4	Monday 29.3
9	Bed Time	10 pm	10.30 pm	11 pm	10.30 pm	11 pm	11 pm	10.30 pm
10	Wake-up Time	5 am	5 am	4.30 am	5 am	5 am	5 am	5 am
11	Time spent in Bed initially trying to sleep after lying down	30 min	15 min	10 min	45 min	15 min	20 min	30 min
12	Sleep Breaks number (duration)	one 2.30 am 1½ hr	one 3.40 am didn't sleep after then	3 am didn't sleep later	One 4 am didn't sleep	one 4.10 am	one 4.30 am didn't sleep later	Two 1.30 Am 1 hr 3.45 am
13	Quality of Sleep & Other Comments	Not good	ok	Not good	ok	ok	ok	Not good
14	Overall rating your sleep out of 10 (if 0 is no sleep and 10 is life best sleep)	3.5	4.5	3.5	4.5	5	5.5	3.5
15	Total sleep Hours	5½ hr	5½ hr	4½ hr	6 hr	5 hr	6½ hr	4½ hr

Figures 17.1–17.14 (Continued)

Sr. No.	Day (Pl add Date)	Monday 12/7	Tuesday 13/7	Wednesday 14/7	Thursday 15/7	Friday 9/7	Saturday 10/7	Sunday 11/7
1	Exercise (type and duration)	walk 1 hr	walk 45 min	walk 1 hr	walk 1½ hr	walk 1 hr	—	walk 1½ hr
2	Naps (time and duration)	—	1½ hr 3-4.30 pm	45 min 2-2.45	—	30 min 1-1.30	—	1 hr 2-30 pm
3	Alcohol (number of pegs)	—	—	—	—	—	—	—
4	Tea & Coffe (number of cups & last)	3 cups last at 5.30 pm	2 cups last at 6pm	3 ½ last at 6.30pm	2 ½ last at 5 pm	3 cups last at 6pm	3 cups last at 5pm	2½ cup last at 4.30 pm
5	Feelings	Good	Good	Good	Good	Good	Good	OK
6	Food & Drink (time of meals)	lunch 1 pm Dinner 8pm	lunch 1.30 pm Dinner 9pm	lunch 1.30pm Dinner 7.45pm	lunch 12.30pm Dinner 10pm	lunch 12.30 pm Dinner 8pm	lunch 1pm Dinner 9pm	lunch 2pm Dinner 8.30pm
7	Medications or sleep Aids	Hypertension Diabetes	Hypertension Diabetes	Hypertension Diabetes	Hypertension Diabetes	Hypertension Diabetes	Hypertension Diabetes	Hypertension Diabetes
8	Bedtime Routine	TV 9 pm (one hour) yoga nidna 60	100	TV 8.30 pm (one hour) 130/77 yoga nidna 65	100	— 128/77	TV 9 pm (one hour) yoga nidna 60	100	TV 9pm (one hour) yoga nidna 68	100	TV 9pm (one hour) 5.30 125/35 yoga nidna 70 / 100	TV 7pm (one hour) 128/78 yoga nidna 65	100

		Tuesday 13/7	Wednesday 14/7	Thursday 15/7	Friday 9/7	Saturday 10/7	Sunday 11/7	Monday 12/7
9	Bed Time	10.30pm	10 pm	11 pm	9.45 pm	10.30pm	10.30pm	10 pm
10	Wake-up Time	5 am	5 am	4.30 am	5 am	5 am	5 am	5 am
11	Time spent in Bed initially trying to sleep after lying down	15 min	10 min approx	10 min	15 min approx	20 min approx	10 min	10 min
12	Sleep Breaks number (duration)	Nil	Nil	1 4.30am	1 4.15 am didn't sleep after that	Nil	Nil	one 2 am approx 1 hr
13	Quality of Sleep & Other Comments	Good	Good	Good	Good	Good	Good	ok
14	Overall rating your sleep out of 10 (if 0 is no sleep and 10 is life best sleep)	7/10	7	7	6.5	6.5	7	6
15	Total sleep Hours	approx 7.5	7 hr 45 min	7 hr	approx 7 hr 15 min	6 hr	7.5	6 hr approx

Figures 17.1–17.14 (Continued)

Sr. No.	Day (Pl add Date)	Monday 20 17	Tuesday 21/7	Wednesday 22/7	Thursday 16/7	Friday 17/7	Saturday 18/7	Sunday 17/7
1	Exercise (type and duration)	1 1/2 hr	45min	1 hr	—		—	4 1/2 hr
2	Naps (time and duration)	30 min 3 - 3.30	45 min 3.30 - 4.45 pm	1 1/2 hr 2 - 3.30 pm			1 hr 3 - 4 pm	45 min
3	Alcohol (number of pegs)	—	—	—	—		—	—
4	Tea & Coffe (number of cups & last	3 cups last cd 5.30 pm	2 1/2 cups	3 1/2 last cd 5.30 pm	2 1/2 cups	way out of Town	3 cups	3 cups last cd 5 pm
5	Feelings	Good	Good	Good	Good		Good	Good
6	Food & Drink (time of meals)	lunch 1.30 Dinner - 2 pm	lunch - 1 pm Dinner 9 pm	lunch - 1.30 pm Dinner 8.30 pm	lunch - 2 pm Dinner 9 pm		lunch . 1 pm Dinner 8.30 pm	lunch 2.30 pm Dinner 9 pm
7	Medications or sleep Aids	Hypertensi on Diabetes	Hypertensi on Diabetes	Hypertensi on Diabetes	Hyperten. sion Diabetes		Hyperten. sion Diabetes	Hyperten slon Diabetes
8	Bedtime Routine	TV 8.30 pm (1 hour)	TV 9.30 pm (1 hour)	TV 9 pm (1 hour)	TV 8.30 pm (1 hour)		TV 9 pm (1 hour)	TV 10 pm (1 hour)
		128/82	131/81 yoga nidna 65/100	130/82 yoga nidna 70/100	119/83 yoga nidna 65/100		117/77 yoga nidna 60/100	118/80 yoga nidna 55/100

		Tuesday 21/7	Wednesday 22/7	Thursday 16/7	Friday 17/7	Saturday 18/7	Sunday 19/7	Monday 20/7
9	Bed Time	10.15 pm	10.45 pm	10.45 pm		11. pm	11 pm	11 pm
10	Wake -up Time	5 am	5 am	5 am		5 am	5 am	5 am
11	Time spent in Bed initially trying to sleep after lying down	10 min	approx 15 min	approx 10-15min		approx 10 min	10-15 min	10 - 15 min
12	Sleep Breaks number (duration)	—	—	one 4 am 15 min		—	one 2 am approx 30-40 min	one 4.30 am
13	Quality of Sleep & Other Comments	Good	Good	ok		Good	ok	Good
14	Overall rating your sleep out of 10 (if 0 is no sleep and 10 is life best sleep)	7/10	7	6.5		7	6	6.5
15	Total sleep Hours	7 hrs 45 min approx	7.5 hrs approx	5.5 hrs approx		7 hrs	6 1/2 hrs approx	6 1/2 hrs

Figures 17.1–17.14 (Continued)

as there was marked reduction in SOL. SOL was less than 30 minutes for most days of the week. Yoga nidra subjective effectiveness score was 60–75%. The patient documented his feelings as "Ok" and "better." Naps were now in the early afternoon.

- 05 Apr–18 Apr 2021: The patient stabilizes further.
- 09–22 Jul 2021: Review the sleep diary in Figures 17.11–17.14, which shows both SOL and WASO less than 30 minutes for most days of the week. Patient continued to feel better, and the subjective quality of sleep was also better.

The specific goals were to improve sleep quality, reduce WASO and SOL, and set the nap time to best suit the patient. The preceding pages of the temporal sleep diary in a case of chronic insomnia shows the intervention effects sequentially. With intermittent sleep diaries over a long period of time, the physician also comes to know the problem areas that require review regularly. For example, in this case, the sleep maintenance and the nap habits require close supervision. Repeatedly emphasizing the role of a short nap earlier in the day rather than in the evening is important in this case.

CONCLUSION

The sleep diary remains an important tool in assessing the patient. Its efficient use by the patient requires that the physician should be conversant with this simple, cheap, and yet effective tool.

SUGGESTED READING

1. Kryger MH, Roth T, Dement WC, editors. *Principles and Practice of Sleep Medicine*. 5th ed. St. Louis, MO: Elsevier Saunders; 2011. 1723 p.
2. Datta K, Tripathi M, Mallick HN. *Yoga Nidra*: an innovative approach for management of chronic insomnia: a case report. *Sleep Sci Pract*. 2017;1:7. https://doi.org/10.1186/s41606-017-0009-4.

18

Actigraphy: Indications, Procedural Do's and Don'ts, Sample Report

KARUNA DATTA, AND THOMAS JOSEPH

INTRODUCTION

Actigraphy uses a portable monitoring device to record an individual's limb movement over time. Both the occurrence as well as the degree of movement are recorded. This data can then be used in the study of normal sleep as well in the assessment of various sleep problems.

Actigraphy was used in the early 1970s to estimate sleep and wake, and the term "actigraphy" was first coined in a 1978 study by Kripke et al., who also used piezoelectric transducers in the device, which have now become the standard for movement-based measurement. In the 1980s, the first automated scoring algorithm for actigraphy was developed, which demonstrated validity against PSG. Since then, more reliable algorithms and technological advancements have been incorporated into actigraphy.

ACTIGRAPH

Modern actigraphs are small devices that contain a movement detector (accelerometer) and digital memory to store the recorded data. The data are then transferred to a PC, which then analyzes the data using software provided by the manufacturer. Earlier devices used mechanical sensors to detect movement. Presently actigraphs use piezoelectric sensors. They also contain lithium batteries and built-in data storage. Modern actigraphs are small and lightweight and don't cause much patient discomfort. They can be placed on the wrist, ankle, or waist. For sleep studies, the subject usually wears the actigraph on the wrist of the non-dominant hand.

Some actigraphs have the capability to record additional parameters like temperature of skin, room noise, and light levels. Another feature that is commonly found in actigraphs is a button that can be pressed by the individual to note various events like lights on/off, bedtime, and other events. Here are some considerations when choosing an actigraphy:

- The accelerometer should be validated to assess sleep. It should have capability for data collection in either time above threshold, digital integration mode, or any such software.
- Product dimensions need to be considered for weight, especially when infants and children are to be assessed.
- Event marker button
- Built-in light sensor
- The battery should be able to record data continuously, preferably for 14 days.
- Data storage should be protected against loss of data even if the battery fails
- Availability of customer support for the device and software is important.

PRINCIPLE

Actigraphy involves the direct measurement of movement and indirect assessment of sleep using specific algorithms. During sleep, there is little movement, whereas a periodic increase in movement occurs during wake. Movement is sampled many times each second, and this is usually stored in epochs of 1 minute duration. The data thus obtained are viewed in the software, checked for errors, and then analyzed to determine whether the subject is in sleep or wake. The data is digitized by the software and scored as wake/sleep by automated computer algorithms that can vary depending on the manufacturer/software.

Digitization of data can be done by three methods: (1) time above threshold (TAT), which uses the duration that the activity crosses a defined threshold in each epoch; (2) zero crossing mode (ZCM), which measures the number of times the signal crosses zero in each epoch; and (3) digital integration mode (DIM), which computes the area under the curve. Some actigraphs can use more than one of these methods.

Sleep estimation algorithms, also called sleep scoring functions, use the movement data

collected by the actigraph (activity counts) during each 1 minute epoch and transforms it into a sleep score, which can have a binary value of 0 (wake) or 1 (sleep). Various validated sleep estimation algorithms depend on factors like the make of the device, age of study population, epoch length, etc. The Cole–Kripke algorithm and the University of California, San Diego (UCSD) scoring algorithm are commonly used algorithms.

The following are the common parameters obtained from the data:

- Total duration of sleep
- Proportion of time in "sleep"
- Total duration of wake
- Proportion of time in "wake"
- Number of wake episodes
- Duration between wake episodes
- Time taken for onset of sleep

PROCEDURE

Before the Test

Before the test, a complete history should be taken, and a physical examination of the patient should be carried out. The history should include sleep history, medication history, and history of any past or present injury/illness. In addition, sleep questionnaires can be used to aid in the assessment of sleep.

The test procedure should be explained to the patient, and an informed consent should be taken. The patient should also be educated about the do's and don'ts and precautions in advance.

The Actigraph battery should be kept fully charged in advance. Following this, the actigraph must be set up to initialize data collection. For this, the device is connected to a computer usually via USB or Bluetooth. In the software provided by the manufacturer, the various study parameters and patient particulars are entered. This includes the start and end times for the data collection. Recording is usually carried out for a duration of 7–14 days as both weekday and weekend sleep patterns can be obtained. The data collection can be started immediately or at a specified time in the future. This helps in conserving battery life and storage of the device.

TEST PROCEDURE

The patient wears the device, usually on the non-dominant wrist, and starts the recording on the device. In infants and toddlers, the actigraph is usually attached to the ankle. The device should fit snugly and should be neither too loose nor too tight.

The patient is also asked to keep a sleep diary for the duration of the study. The following events should be mentioned in the sleep diary (details on how to complete a sleep diary are given in Chapter 17):

- Bedtime
- Time taken by the subject to fall asleep after deciding to sleep
- Any sleep breaks
- Wake-up time
- Time at which subject was out of the bed
- Daytime naps
- Time that the actigraph was removed and worn again
- Any other situations that could have interfered with sleep—illness, travel, etc.

In addition, the subject is instructed to press the event marker button on the actigraph during any nighttime awakenings in addition to the events just listed.

Precautions

- The battery should be fully charged in advance and checked before initializing the recording.
- If the recording duration is more than a week, the data can be downloaded every week to prevent loss of data in case a battery problem is suspected.
- For devices with a light sensor, the subject should be instructed to ensure that it is not covered by the sleeve or any part of clothing.
- The device and sensors should be checked periodically to determine if calibration is required.
- If the subject's skin is sensitive, the actigraph can be taken off for a short duration daily to avoid pressure sores. The same is logged in the sleep diary.
- If the device is removed during the duration of the recording, the subject is instructed to put it back on the same wrist.

- The subject should be instructed to not get the device wet if it is not water resistant. To be on the safe side, the instrument should be kept from being wet even if it is water resistant.

ANALYSIS AND INTERPRETATION

The actigraphy recording can be uploaded and viewed on a laptop or computer immediately after the actigraph is taken off the wrist. The sleep diary, along with event markers, are used to aid in editing the data. Data corresponding to periods toward the start and finish of the recording when the actigraph was not worn by the subject are deleted. If the device has been removed for any activity, e.g., bathing, exercise, etc., and the same is mentioned in the sleep diary, the period is manually scored as wake. In case of any uncertainty, the period should be marked as missing data or deleted to prevent it from being automatically scored as sleep. Also look for any aberrant movements in the recording, which should raise suspicion of a device error. In that case, the corresponding part of the data should be omitted from the analysis.

The actigraph usually comes with software that can be used for scoring rest/activity and identifying the status as sleep or wake. One such actigraphy template represented pictorially is shown in Figure 18.1, wherein activity, light, and sleep/wake are marked. These reports generated by software can be exported as an Excel file or as a detailed report for in-depth analysis.

EVIDENCE

The American Academy of Sleep Medicine (AASM) releases clinical practice guidelines on the use of actigraphy in sleep disorders based on available evidence. The recommendations are classified as Strong and Conditional. Strong recommendations are meant to be followed for most patients, while Conditional recommendations should be implemented based on clinical judgment on a case-to-case basis.

Studies have compared actigraphy against polysomnography (PSG), which is considered the gold standard in sleep assessment. In individuals who do not have any sleep abnormalities, the total duration of sleep obtained using actigraphy had good correlation when compared to polysomnography.

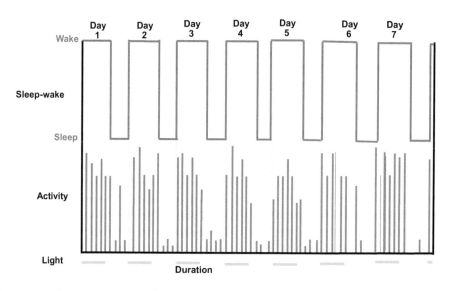

Figure 18.1 Pictorial representation of actigraphy record showing periods of sleep and wake, light, and activity over 7 days.

Actigraphy estimates of sleep efficiency and wake after sleep onset were also found to be useful. However, time to sleep onset obtained by actigraphy had lower consistency, and, in general, correlations were found to be reduced in severely disturbed sleep. Good correlation between actigraphy and PSG were also obtained in studies involving infants and children. In subjects with severe sleep apnea and those on antidepressants, the correlation was lower compared to PSG.

Various factors like the model of the actigraph, the population under study, the device settings, and the algorithm employed can influence the total sleep duration obtained using actigraphy. Also, actigraphy may not correlate well with PSG at each minute, especially in cases of disturbed sleep. Variation has also been noted between different devices; thus, the investigator has to be cautious when comparing results from studies using different devices. Reliability studies are required for each model of actigraph and for the specific population group being studied.

APPLICATIONS

Actigraphy is a reliable tool in the assessment of sleep in normal populations. However, it may not be reliable in many sleep disorders. AASM has given conditional recommendations for the use of actigraphy in the assessment of following conditions:

- Insomnia disorder (in adult patients to estimate sleep parameters and in pediatric patients for assessment)
- Circadian rhythm sleep-wake disorder (in adults and pediatric patients)
- To estimate total sleep time (TST) integrated with home sleep apnea test devices, in the evaluation of patients suspected to have sleep disordered breathing
- Monitoring total duration of sleep before a Multiple Sleep Latency Test in adult and pediatric patients in whom a central disorder of hypersomnolence is suspected—to ensure adequate sleep prior to testing
- Insufficient sleep syndrome-to estimate TST

In addition, a strong recommendation to *not use* actigraphy as a monitoring device for movements in the diagnosis of periodic limb movement disorder has been given.

Actigraphy is also useful for studying the effects of treatment due to its ability to identify changes in sleep patterns over time. In addition, it can be used during follow-up assessments during the course of treatment and also to screen patients for sleep problems.

The additional parameters recorded by the actigraph can be useful in specific conditions. Ambient light measurements comprising the amount and duration of light exposure are useful in studying advanced and delayed sleep-wake phase disorders. This can also aid in the development of a treatment plan. Some actigraphs have a built-in microphone to detect snoring, and some can measure skin temperature, which is useful in the study of circadian rhythm. Actigraphy with extended EEG, EMG, and EOG capability, such that objective scoring of stages is possible, is also available for commercial use. Actigraphy is also available with extended ECG recording capability.

Actigraphy can be used in research and has been used in many cohort studies of the relation between sleep and various health parameters. The relatively low cost, better subject compliance, and ease of use make actigraphy a useful tool in large population studies. Study areas have included the relationship of sleep with outcomes such as impaired cognition, propensity for falls, reduced exercise performance, risk of obesity, and serum cholesterol levels. One such study done in an elite archer using actigraphy with EEG module is placed in suggested reading for those interested.

COMPARISON WITH SMARTWATCHES AND SMARTPHONE-BASED SLEEP APPLICATIONS

Various commercially available devices are marketed as having the capability to assess sleep. These include smartphone applications that make use of the accelerometer in the device and smartwatches such as Fitbit and Apple watch worn on the wrist. Some smartwatches use accelerometers similar to the ones used in actigraphy. In addition, they are more widely available, cheaper, and the results are easy to interpret. While smartphones may not accurately depict sleep, few smartwatches have given results comparable to actigraphy. Some of these devices may be a good start for monitoring sleep in otherwise healthy people, but there is a need to check the validation of the device before use. For research, most of these devices don't provide access to the raw data for more in-depth analysis.

Sleep applications can draw from multiple modalities that include both built-in and external sensors and questionnaires. Hence, they can provide more detailed analysis, including sleep stages. However, most of such applications are not scientifically validated and give results in formats that are difficult to convert to standard sleep parameters. Some studies have shown that they have comparable accuracy to actigraphy in sleep-wake discrimination. In addition, there are apps specifically designed to detect snoring/OSA, which have specific algorithms.

Such devices and applications would require more validation studies before they can be used for the clinical assessment of sleep.

ADVANTAGES

While actigraphy cannot be a substitute for PSG, it has many advantages, thus making it a useful tool in a sleep medicine physician's arsenal. They include:

- Convenient and low patient burden, less invasive than PSG.
- Relatively low cost.
- Data that are continuous and objective in contrast to a sleep diary, which gives discrete and subjective data.
- Elimination of laboratory effects as the subjects can sleep in their own homes.
- Longitudinal assessment capability as the device can be worn 24 hours/day for extended durations.
- Ability to be used to assess treatment response and in follow-up.
- More reliable estimates of sleep as data are collected over multiple nights.
- In pediatric populations, reduction of the caregiver's burden and minimization of issues of compliance to sleep logs by the child/caregiver, who can often be unreliable.

LIMITATIONS

- Although cheaper than PSG, actigraphy is still costlier when compared to sleep diaries or sleep questionnaires.
- Actigraphy is currently not reliable enough to be recommended as a stand-alone method for the diagnosis of a sleep disorder.

- While actigraphy in its usual form can distinguish between wake and sleep, it has not been validated for measuring sleep stages.
- Validity is limited in the estimation of sleep onset latency and daytime sleeping.
- Since it can incorrectly classify a subject who is awake but lying motionless as asleep, actigraphy can overestimate TST and thus underestimate the sleep disturbance. This is especially important in hospitalized and bed-bound individuals as they may not have much activity while awake.
- Although no major adverse effects are associated with the use of actigraphy, some patients may develop a minor skin irritation, and few may have difficulty sleeping because of wearing the actigraphy watch.

CONCLUSION

Actigraphy is an easy-to-use technique for assessment and evaluation in the management of sleep disorders. It has many advantages over an overnight polysomnography and should be used where recommended. However, relying on it totally where an overnight polysomnography is indicated might mislead the physician. Actigraphy devices with built-in features may be an option to explore. Actigraphy remains an important tool in outlying areas where overnight polysomnography is not available.

SUGGESTED READING

1. Smith MT, McCrae CS, Cheung J, Martin JL, Harrod CG, Heald JL, Carden KA. Use of actigraphy for the evaluation of sleep disorders and circadian rhythm sleep-wake disorders: an American Academy of Sleep Medicine clinical practice guideline. *J Clin Sleep Med.* 2018;14(7):1231–1237.
2. Datta K, Kumar A, Sekar C. Enhancement of performance in an elite archer after nonpharmacological intervention to improve sleep. *Med J Armed Forces India.* 2020;76(3):338–341. http://doi.org/10.1016/j.mjafi.2018.06.010.

19

Home Sleep Apnea Testing

DEEPAK SHRIVASTAVA

APPROVAL OF HOME SLEEP TESTING BY CMS

In 2007, the Agency for Healthcare Research and Quality published a landmark article reassessing the state of the art in our understanding of home-based diagnostics for sleep apnea. This analysis was an evidence-based prelude to the 2007 Centers for Medicare & Medicaid Services (CMS) reexamination of the evidence for home sleep apnea testing, which led to its decision in 2008 to allow home sleep apnea testing results to be used for the provision of CPAP therapy for sleep apnea.

With regard to home sleep apnea testing (HSAT), when combined with clinical history, for many forms of home sleep apnea technology currently in existence, there was no conclusive evidence that it was substantially better or substantially worse than traditional PSG for making a diagnosis of OSA. Their decision has allowed for type 3, type 2, and type 1 monitors to be more or less equivalent for allowing a diagnosis of sleep apnea in order to provide CPAP therapy. Level 4 monitors were excluded from this approval. However, the final national coverage determination (NCD) developed a category called level 4 with three channels that are covered by CMS.

TYPES OF HSAT MONITORS

Home sleep apnea monitors are classified based on the number and complexity of the signal that can be recorded.

Type 1: This is the standard in-lab polysomnography testing.

Type 2: This is a miniature, portable, but comprehensive polysomnographic testing unit with the similar setup to the type 1 in-lab test that can be performed in other settings than the sleep laboratory.

Type 3: Cardiopulmonary symptoms are recorded by a minimum of 4 signals that include monitoring of the airflow at the nose and mouth, respiratory effort by the basal attributes, measurements of the heart rate, and pulse oximetry. This is the most common type of the HSAT in current use.

Type 4: This type of device records one or two sleep parameters like a pulse oximetry or airflow. Type 4 with three channels is a new addition to the accepted classification because it was used in the CMS National Coverage Determination (NCD) to distinguish different type 4 monitors. Recently according to the CMS guidance, 3 channels

DOI: 10.1201/9781003093381-22

are included: pulse oximetry, respiratory effort monitoring, and measurement of airflow.

WatchPAT: This monitoring device is based on physiologic signal change recordings of peripheral arterial tonometry that has proven to be an accurate surrogate measure for airflow and respiratory-effort-defined sleep disordered breathing devices. The national CMS decision includes the WatchPAT (Itamar Medical, Framingham, MA) as an approved device for the home diagnosis of OSA. At present, Medicare contractors are not including durable medical equipment (DME) on the list of approved methods for diagnosing OSA for the provision of continuous positive airway pressure (CPAP) therapy.

Type 2 Monitors

Advantages

- Ability to record full montage of multiple channels
- Flexibility of selecting signal type
- Equally comprehensive as type 1 study
- Standard sleep analysis software of a type 1 polysomnography used
- Movable to patient location
- Good experience and track record

Disadvantages

- Technician hookup
- Expensive
- Inability of correcting loss of signal at night in case of malfunction

Type 3 Monitors

Advantages

- Easy for patients and their caregivers to use
- Much cheaper than Type 1 and 2 studies
- Movable or mailable to patient location
- Limited to only four recording channels

Disadvantages

- Only few parameters are recorded with the risk of missed information
- Inability of correcting loss of signal at night in case of malfunction
- Many machines can autoscore; a trained technician is needed for evaluation of the information.

Type 4 monitors

Advantages

- As portable as type 3 equipment
- Much cheaper than types 1, 2, and 3 studies
- Easy for patients and their caregivers to use
- Records only core signals

Disadvantages

- Probably a screening tool as it does not capture all the information needed to make a good diagnosis
- Inability of correcting loss of signal at night in case of malfunction

WHEN HOME SLEEP TESTING IS NOT RECOMMENDED

Congestive heart failure
COPD
Hypoventilation
Prior surgery for sleep apnea
Other severe systemic illnesses

While home sleep testing is not recommended for mild pretest probability of obstructive sleep apnea, it is a reasonable choice for moderate to severe pretest probability of OSA. In order to establish pretest probability, the STOP-BANG Questionnaire can be used:

- **S**noring
- **T**iredness, fatigue, or sleepiness during daytime
- **O**bservation by others witnessing breathing cessation
- **P**ressure (hypertension)
- **B**MI over 35
- **A**ge more than 50
- **N**eck circumference 17 inches (40 cm)
- **G**ender (more prevalent in males)

A total score of 5 or higher indicates high probability of moderate to severe obstructive sleep apnea. In that case, home sleep testing may be appropriate.

In addition, many comorbid conditions including chronic pulmonary disease, CHF, hypoventilation, movement disorders of sleep, parasomnias, and central sleep apnea similar other clinical symptoms are contraindications for the home sleep test. The main reason for this recommendation is that HST use is not validated in this patient subset, and the results may be inconclusive. A complete, full-night-in-the-lab polysomnography is recommended in such cases.

COMMONLY USED HOME SLEEP TEST DEVICE OVERVIEW

All level 3 devices measure airflow at the mouth and nose, respiratory effort, pulse oximetry, heart rate, and the patient's body position. These are validated devices and are moderately expensive. Device recording needs a moderate amount of technician time for scoring.

The representative tracings in Figure 19.1 are an example of a typical type 3 device recording output. From top to bottom, the channels represent episodes of oxygen desaturation, heart rate, and airflow tracings with episodes of apnea in the cessation of effort as shown in Figures 19.2 and 19.3.

The computer software allows changing the resolution of the screen and therefore a compressed representative display of all the recorded channels can be examined for breathing and airway obstruction patterns.

The level 4 device measures the airflow and oximetry only. In general, it shows accuracy in detecting severe OSA. Given the low number of monitored channels, it is relatively expensive and requires limited technician time for scoring. The report format is similar to the type 3 HST study.

A rather new technology records and displays changes in peripheral arterial tonometry (PAT). Peripheral arterial tone is a measurement of sympathetic activity. The PAT signal is a marker for obstructive apneas and hypoxia events. This device is moderately expensive. However, it only needs minimal to no technician time for scoring.

Many type 2 machines are validated for collection of sleep data outside the sleep center and at the patient's home. They record and project the airflow changes, EEG findings, and corresponding variations in oximetry.

HST technology is limited to sleep disordered breathing and cannot be used for other non-breathing-related sleep disorders. There is a risk of an incomplete assessment of sleep disordered breathing due to the unattended setting. While starting the home sleep testing program, a needs assessment regarding the choice of the device is highly recommended. The device should be simple to use, have accuracy in the leads, and automatically report the ability, and it is often scoring. The total number of channels can be compared with the cost and options. The new machine should be compatible with the existing PSG software.

The location of the setup and use of home sleep testing is important. Home setup can potentially expose technologists to high-risk settings. The home setup, however, is more likely to have sensors applied accurately. Other practical issues include attaching the equipment to the patient in the lab or providing training for home attachment and activation of the device. One must anticipate and

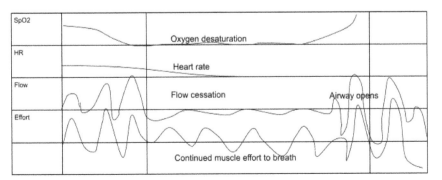

Illustration by: Deepak Shrivastava, MD

Figure 19.1 (SpO$_2$ = oxygen saturation, HR = heart rate, flow = airflow, effort = movement of the chest belt). The tracings show episodes of obstructive sleep apnea with oxygen desaturation.

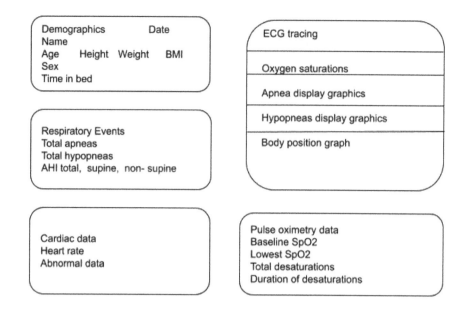

Schematic layout of a level 3 HST: Illustration by: Deepak Shrivastava, MD

Figure 19.2 Typical layout of the type 3 HST report displays demographic information, respiratory and cardiac events in the left panels and graphic display of heart rate, oxygen saturation, obstructive events, and hypopneic events, as well as body position and pulse oximetry data, in the right panel.

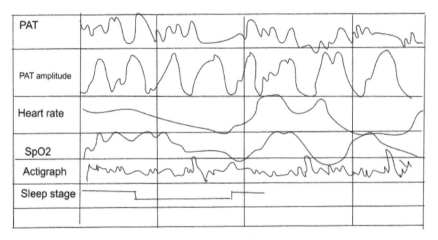

Illustration by: Deepak Shrivastava, MD

Figure 19.3 Pictorial representation of traces of PAT, heart rate, oxygen saturation, and actigraph (PAT = arterial pulse tonometry, PAT amplitude = changes in the tone of the arterial pulse, pulse rate = heart rate, SpO$_2$ = oxygen saturation, actigraph = movement recording, WT 100 = sleep stages).

be flexible regarding the variability in the patient's skills and inability to hook up the machine.

The American Academy of Sleep Medicine, in its position statement in 2020, suggests that the test must be recommended and ordered by a health care provider for the diagnosis of sleep disordered breathing. The recorded data in its original form from the portable device are reviewed and interpreted by a board-certified or board-eligible sleep physician. Home sleep testing is used for the diagnosis of OSA in adult patients who do not have significant cardiovascular or neuromuscular disease. Home sleep study is usually cost-effective and cheaper compared to a complete polysomnography.

DISCLAIMER

This chapter does not review all the products that may be available in a certain geographic area. The reader is encouraged to explore the local availability of approved products and review their features. The author does not have any product preferences or commercial interest in any of the available products.

SUGGESTED READING

1. Rosen IM, Kirsch DB, Chervin RD, Carden KA, Ramar K, Aurora RN, Kristo DA, Malhotra RK, Martin JL, Olson EJ, Rosen CL, Rowley JA. American Academy of Sleep Medicine Board of Directors. Clinical use of a home sleep apnea test: an American Academy of Sleep Medicine position statement. *J Clin Sleep Med.* 2017;13(10):1205–1207.

2. Zou D, et al. Validation of a portable monitoring device for sleep apnea diagnosis in a population based cohort using synchronized home polysomnography. *SLEEP.* 2006;29(3):367–374.

3. Yalamanchali S, Farajian V, Hamilton C, Pott TR, Samuelson CG, Friedman M. Diagnosis of obstructive sleep apnea by peripheral arterial tonometry: meta-analysis. *JAMA Otolaryngol Head Neck Surg.* 2013;139(12):1343–1350.

4. Hedner J, et al. A novel adaptive wrist actigraphy algorithm for sleep-wake assessment in sleep apnea patients. *SLEEP.* 2004;27(8):1560–1566.

20

Polysomnography I: Detail with Indications, Hookup Procedure, Do's and Don'ts

KARUNA DATTA

INTRODUCTION

Polysomnography is a recording of multiple physiological variables to study the physiological changes that occur in sleep and to correlate them to the various stages of sleep. Essentially the digital polysomnography records the various phases of sleep-wake (wake, REM, and NREM sleep); picks up artifacts; analyzes the ECG for rate, rhythm, heart rate variability (if possible), pulse saturations; analyzes respiratory movements and oronasal airflow to check for apnea, types of apnea (obstructive or central, hypopnea, respiratory-event-related arousal [RERA], and noninvasive blood pressure using pulse transit time and ECG

[if possible]); and abnormal movements from the EMG. It then correlates these to one another and to various stages of sleep. Here, we discuss this test to simplify the concept and provide the guidelines available.

HISTORY

In the early twentieth century, emerging evidence appeared regarding the role of the EEG in psychology and psychiatry, and recordings of these signals were conducted for research. In 1928, Hans Berger, a German psychiatrist, recorded electrical activity of the human brain. He called these recordings 'electroencephalograms,' known today as EEG.

DOI: 10.1201/9781003093381-23

It was also found that EEG recordings showed a marked difference in the sleep and wake states. Characterization of human sleep occurred in 1937, when Davis et al. at Harvard University studied sleep brain wave patterns and characterized human sleep. High-amplitude low-frequency slow waves and spindles characterized human sleep, and low-amplitude high-frequency beta waves and alpha rhythm were used for characterization of wakefulness. The unitary concept of sleep prevailed until Eugene Aserinsky, a graduate student of Kleitman in 1952, was assigned the job to observe eye movements in infants and later also in adults while asleep.

Following this, a method of electrooculography (EOG) for continuously measuring eye movements was devised. Several bursts of potential changes on EOG were recorded during sleep, and they were quite different from the slow movements at sleep onset. The seminal paper in 1953 by Aserinsky and Kleitman was a breakthrough in sleep research as the duality of sleep—REM and non-REM or NREM came into being. Whole-night recordings were still not done in order to conserve paper as there was a paucity of funds, but in 1959, motivated by Aserinsky's results, Dement and Kleitman recorded 126 full-night recordings with 33 subjects and, with the help of EEG patterns, scored the paper recordings in their entirety. When the scoring was complete, they correlated the patterns and found that these patterns occurred repeatedly at an interval of approximately 90–110 minutes while the subject was asleep. A cyclical nature was determined, and NREM and REM percentages of the total sleep time were also found. The suppression of muscle potentials during REM sleep in cats was studied by Michel Jouvet. In the 1960s, Hodes and Dement worked on the H reflex in humans and found the complete suppression of H reflex during REM sleep, and the importance of electromyography during sleep recording was realized.

Thus, for delineating the different stages of sleep and distinguishing them from wake, EEG, EOG, and EMG recordings are essential.

In 1968, Rechtschaffen and Kales propounded sleep staging criteria using EEG, EOG, and EMG. Jerome Holland at Stanford University coined the term "polysomnography" in 1974 and added cardiac and respiratory sensors to the EEG, EOG, and EMG.

WHAT IS POLYSOMNOGRAPHY?

Polysomnography is the recording of various biological signals during sleep. These signals provide different information regarding the physiological variables. This information helps in scoring sleep or in monitoring physiology during sleep: for example, heart rate information from ECG; airflow trace from an oronasal thermistor; respiratory effort from thoracic and abdominal effort belts, etc. In other words, polysomnography is a multichannel record designed to document a variety of physiological activities during sleep.

MONTAGE AND SENSORS

A standard PSG montage requires an EEG, EMG, ECG, oronasal thermistor, nasal cannula, limb leads, pulse oximeter, respiratory effort belts, body position sensor, and snoring sensor. A PAP device flow may be required where CPAP would be used during the study for titrations. Recommended filter settings and sampling rates for the proper acquisition of the data from various sensors are required. Most of the digital acquisition machines follow AASM guidelines, and compliance should be ensured in the montage before starting the study. The montage is completed with the location of EEG channels and marking the location of ground and reference electrodes.

CONDUCT OF PSG

Indications

1. PSG is not indicated to diagnose insomnia alone but it is indicated in case there is a clinical suspicion of coexisting sleep disorder like CRSWD, OSA or PLMD.

2. Diagnosis of OSA, central sleep apnea, other sleep-related breathing disorders; central causes of hypersomnolence, narcolepsy, parasomnias, PLMD, and sleep-related movement disorders when suspected clinically either alone or in combination with another sleep disorder even with bruxism or insomnia.

3. Cases of sleep disorders on treatment, not responding to therapy or showing emergence of new symptoms; or suspicion of development of any other coexisting disorder. PSG is indicated in:

- OSA on treatment with CPAP with newly diagnosed stroke; arrythmias especially at night or increases in blood pressure for the first time or in a hypertensive, despite treatment with antihypertensives.
- Insomnia on a nonpharmacological approach using cognitive behavioral therapy for insomnia (CBTI) and now not responding or refractory; or worsening of the disease despite continuation of treatment.
- Circadian rhythm sleep-wake disorder (CRSWD) with recent comorbidities—endocrinal, cardiovascular, neurological, or metabolic—in a case of a shift worker.
- CRSWD with clinical suspicion of another sleep disorder or to diagnose non-24-hour CRSWD, irregular sleep-wake disorder.
- NREM or REM parasomnia not responding to or deteriorating despite treatment, clinical suspicion to rule out seizures; coexisting sleep disorder; emergence of new comorbidity of cardiovascular, neurological, endocrinal, or metabolic disorder; to rule out OSA, central sleep apnea, mixed sleep apnea, RERA, OSAS.
- Clinical suspicion of PLMD.

3. Follow-up PSG in adults is indicated when, despite PAP therapy, symptoms start to recur, and response to PAP needs to be assessed; weight gain or loss after PAP therapy starts; recent change in blood pressure, arrythmias at night, TIA/stroke despite being on PAP (required to reassess the sleep-related hypoxemia).

4. PSG in children is indicated to ascertain the diagnosis of PLMD once clinical suspicion is present. Similarly, when NREM parasomnias, epilepsy, nocturnal enuresis is present, screening for OSA or PLMD are required, PSG is indicated.

5. PSG is required with extended montage in children with dangerously injurious parasomnia in order to rule out sleep-related epilepsy.

6. PSG is indicated in children with OSAS before undergoing adenotonsillectomy as treatment for OSAS and after adenotonsillectomy if residual symptoms are clinically suspected to be present.

7. PSG in children is indicated when a diagnosis is to be ascertained after clinical suspicion of

OSAS; PAP titration for OSAS; in follow-up in chronic PAP for OSAS when symptoms reoccur, for reassessment of the child for a change in the requirement of pressures in PAP due to child growth and anticipated change in size.

8. In an infant for ascertaining a diagnosis with clinical suspicion of primary sleep apnea of infancy, if the infant with OSAS has had an apparent life-threatening event.

9. In a child after rapid maxillary expansion, oral appliance therapy to evaluate the residual symptoms or treatment.

10. PSG can be done in children on noninvasive positive pressure ventilation for other SRBD, before decannulation after tracheostomy for SRBD; also, in SRBD cases given suspicion of other disorders like asthma, cystic fibrosis, chronic hypoventilation, pulmonary hypertension, etc.

PSG is not indicated for establishing a diagnosis of insomnia, sleep deprivation, shift work disorder, DSWPD, ASWPD, jet lag syndrome alone. It is not recommended for sleep-related bruxism in children. However, if these disorders are suspected with another disorder or if child does not respond with the recommended therapy, PSG is indicated to ascertain the diagnosis.

INSTRUCTIONS TO PATIENT AND FOR LAB

Do's and Don'ts for PSG Night Study

DO'S

Before Starting the Study

1. Switch on AC, and follow all COVID precautions.
2. Fully charge the PSG device.
3. Ensure the wireless device is switched on and connected to PSG device (blue light on both devices).
4. Ensure the router is plugged in and switched on.
5. Ensure that the camera and speaker in the bedroom are switched on.
6. Ensure that the microphone is connected to the USB port of the PC.

7. Verify the details of the subject from the approved list.
8. Make the subject comfortable, explain the procedure, and obtain consent.
9. Once the PSG hookup is completed and initiated through the online mode, check that all signals can be seen on the PC. Check the impedances of all electrodes, and ensure they are less than 5 kΩ.

During the Study

1. Lights off and Lights on should be marked in the software.
2. Video, microphone, and all signals should be working fine.
3. Subject and subject parameters should be constantly monitored.
4. Watch for the following:
   a. Abnormal movements
   b. Reduced or absent breathing
   c. Loss of signal or high impedance in any electrode
   d. Abnormalities in the ECG
   e. Reduced oxygen saturation
5. In case of the loss of signal or high impedance, the technician is to go in quietly and physically check the electrode and reattach it if required. (However, if any one of F3/F4 and C3/C4 and O1/O2, along with the Mastoid electrode of the opposite side, is working fine, then the technician is not required to go in.)
6. In case of apneic episode, the technician should wake the subject up gently.
7. If subject moves out of bed or does any movements that are injury prone, the technician should wake up the subject and accompany her or him back to bed, unless advised not to.
8. In case of any emergency, the medical officer should be promptly informed.

After the Study

1. Disconnect and clean the electrodes with distilled water and dry them before replacement in the box.
2. Ensure that all attached PSG components have been removed and are placed in the bag.
3. Hand over the PSG equipment and keys to the sleep lab and cupboard to the sleep lab staff in the morning.

DON'TS

1. Don't start the study unless all the signals required, including video and audio connections, are working fine and can be viewed online.
2. Avoid unnecessary movements and sounds near the subject.
3. Don't ignore any indications of discomfort or distress made by the subject.
4. Don't leave the subject unattended at any time.
5. Don't leave the sleep lab unattended at any time.

HOOKUP

EEG, EOG, and EMG Channels

The EEG, EOG, and EMG are recorded after placing electrodes on the scalp and skin surfaces. The site is cleaned and properly prepared with skin preparation gel to ensure a good contact such that the electrical impedance is kept at 5000 Ω or less. Scalp electrodes are affixed with electrode conductive paste. Electrode application to identify location is as per the EEG Society's international 10–20 system. A montage using only F3, F4, O1, O2, C3, and C4 positions is used as a standard EEG montage for PSG and referenced to the contralateral mastoid. F3, O1, and C3 are placed as a backup in case the contralateral corresponding side is moved or removed from the scalp during sleep.

EOG channels, one on each side at the outer canthi, are placed, the right EOG electrode 1 cm above and the left electrode 1 cm below the outer canthus. This placement helps to identify both horizontal and vertical movements of the eye.

EMG Channels

A pair of electrodes are placed at the submentalis muscle for recording EMG. One electrode is placed at the midline, 1 cm above the mandible's inferior edge, and is referenced to another one placed 2 cm below and 2 cm to the right (or left) from this reference electrode. Practically at night, if both right and left electrodes are applied, then one of them intends to act as backup in case one of them loses contact with the skin surface.

ECG

Lead II ECG electrodes are placed according to standard criteria and connected to the headbox.

Oronasal Airflow Using Thermistor

For the pressure-based sensor, the nasal pressure cannula is positioned above the upper lip with the cannula protruding slightly into the nostrils.

For the thermistor sensor, the sensor is positioned so that the flexible tabs fit under the nostrils. The tabs are pinched back 90° so that they are comfortable, yet not touching the skin and not protruding into the nostrils. The tabs are bent outward, away from the patient's face. The leads are then draped over the patient's ears, and the inputs are connected into the headbox.

Limb Leads

Respiratory effort belts and pulse oximetry are placed, and the signal is monitored along with the recording of snoring sounds with the microphone sensor placed on the neck.

BIOCALIBRATION

Before starting the study, biocalibration using common instructions is done: for example, types of eye movements (moving up/down; right/left; fast blinks, reading type), grinding teeth, moving legs, taking a deep breath and stopping it, breathing slowly and then rapidly to check flow, pressure and the respiratory effort. The individual is asked to count slowly, and the snoring sensor trace checked. Closing the eyes shows alpha waves at the occipital area in alpha generators and helps identify the alpha block once the individual now opens the eyes. Once the alpha waves are seen, the attenuation of these waves by 50% in an epoch can be kept as a criterion for N1, along with slowly rolling eye movements and the vertex wave. This is important not only to check that the sensors are connected, and acquisition is fine but also to check back on some recording with these markings like eye movements for the type of sleep, etc.

RUNNING THE TEST

Artifact Detection

Artifacts are signals that are extraneous in nature and affect the analysis. A signal that interferes with the analysis of another is also considered an artifact: for example, if an ECG trace is recorded in the EEG trace, ECG is the artifact in the EEG recording. Artifacts may originate either from the patient, e.g., from sweat, an ECG trace in the EEG signal, eye movements trace in the EEG. They may be due to the equipment: e.g., a broken or faulty electrode, improper connection of the lead to the headbox; a sensor not connected at all, etc. Or they may be due to the external factors, such as 50/60 Hz impedance. The common types of artifacts seen during the study are sweat artifacts, ECG trace seen in EEG/EOG trace, movement artifacts, snore artifacts, incorrect filter or gain settings, 60/50 Hz impedance or high impedance, or artifacts emerging because of an electrode popping off the subject.

Recognizing these artifacts is important, and troubleshooting is extremely vital for a clean polysomnography record. At the start of the study, in case an artifact is seen, one can check the montage and its setting, recalibrate the amplifier, and, if still not corrected, try to identify the type of artifact. ECG artifacts in the EEG trace can be simply corrected at the start of the study. In case it is missed, some machines have an option of ECG correction which is done by eliminating the ECG signal from the trace where the artifact is visible. Ideally it should be checked initially and amended at the start of the study by changing the location of the electrode.

At the start of the study, if the tracing appears artifact free, and then, during the study, artifacts appear, adequate trouble shooting is required. Sweat artifacts appear as slow waves and may mimic delta waves. The appearance of these in a few EEG channels and the lack of disappearance even when the stage appears to have changed from N3 to N1/N2/REM/wake in other channels should raise an alarm and help identify the sweat artifact.

Some golden rules for correction of artifacts once identified are as follows:

- If the artifact appears in a channel to which backup is already available, such as the chin EMG, alternate EEG channel, etc., then let the patient sleep and do not try to fix the problem during the study.
- If the artifact is appearing in multiple EEG electrodes, look for a common source: the contralateral mastoid for all common electrodes on one side; the ground electrode if all EEG electrodes are involved, etc. Also look carefully

for whether this artifact in multiple channels is related to the patient behavior, e.g., a snoring artifact, movement artifact, etc.

- If after checking all the wires, electrodes, connections, and ruling out all possible sources of possible sites, one is not able to discern the cause, it is best to make notes during the night when the artifact appears and whether it is related to movement, respiration, sweat, switching off the fan or AC, etc.

SCORING AND REPORTING THE STUDY

Scoring Rules for Staging Sleep

The night record is scored epoch-wise. For sleep staging, a standard 30 second epoch is taken, and each epoch scored as per the recommended criteria of the American Association of Sleep Medicine (AASM). Broad guidelines of scoring the wake and various stages of sleep are discussed next.

- **Wake:** Beta waves or low-amplitude mixed-frequency EEG; reading eye movements, eye blinks, and irregular conjugate eye movements are seen. Alpha waves appear especially at the occipital region when eyes are closed but the individual is awake.
- **NREM:** This type of sleep has four stages: I, II, III and IV. Rechtschaffen and Kales criteria are used for all stages, but as per the AASM guideline, stages III and IV are combined as N3 during the scoring and staging of sleep. The identifying features of each are as follows:
  - N1: Individuals who generate alpha waves on EEG when eyes closed but are awake show more than 50% attenuation of alpha in an epoch, and the EEG now shows low amplitude mixed frequency during N1 sleep. This is accompanied by slow rolling movements in EOG, and there may be a slight reduction in EMG tone as compared to wake. Vertex wave may be seen, which is sharp and of less than 0.5 second duration.
  - N2: N2 sleep is characterized by one or more K-complexes and one and more trains of sleep spindles that are not associated with arousal. EEG remains low amplitude mixed frequency, but

intermittently one sees K-complex and spindles. K-complex is a typical sharp negative, followed by a large positive wave. The entire duration of K-complex is more than 0.5 second and is seen maximally at the frontal location. Spindles are 12–14 Hz waves maximally seen at a central location, and duration is more than 0.5 second.

- An individual in N2 can proceed to N3, may have an arousal or body movements, and slip to stage N1 or wake. The subject may also show REM sleep after N2.
- **N3:** This stage is called the slow wave sleep stage. This comprises both stage III and stage IV. N3 is scored when an epoch shows more than 20% of the epoch with delta waves. Delta waves characteristically are 0.5–4 Hz maximally seen at the central region, and the amplitude of these waves is more than 75 µV.
- **R:** REM sleep is scored when the EEG shows low amplitude high frequency. There is minimal EMG tone seen in the chin EMG as compared to wake and NREM. There are rapid, irregular, sharply peaked conjugate eye movements. Due to the appearance of the EEG being like wake, it is also called paradoxical sleep.

The details on scoring various stages, along with transition from one stage to another, follow AASM guidelines.

Scoring Events

What events should one look for in the polysomnography record, and how should one score them?

While scrolling through the polysomnography epochs, one should look for unusual occurrences like a change in EMG tone, movements, artifacts, arousals, arrhythmias, abnormal behavior, abnormal breathing patterns, etc. For beginners, it is advisable to do the scoring of events after the scoring for staging sleep is done. Some common events are mentioned in brief here. Recent AASM guidelines should be checked for scoring these events in detail.

When Is It an Arousal?

Arousal is a sudden shift in EEG frequency of more than 16 Hz. First, it should be confirmed that they are not spindles. This shift in frequency should be after at least 10 seconds of stable sleep to be called an arousal and should last for at least 3 seconds. If marked during REM, it should have an increase in EMG tone for at least a second. The arousal index is calculated by multiplying 60 with the number of arousals during the record and dividing it by total sleep time (TST).

Whenever an arousal is noted, which is marked automatically by digital polysomnography software, we should ascertain and confirm its presence and then try to find out a cause, if any. For example, is it related to desaturation due to a respiratory problem, apnea, hypopnea, arrhythmia, periodic limb movement, body movements, or is it spontaneous, i.e., without any evident cause?

When Is It a Periodic Limb Movement?

A periodic limb movement is scored when a limb movement is not within 0.5 second (neither preceding nor following the movement) of an apnea, hypopnea, or respiratory-event-related arousal or sleep disordered breathing. An increase of a minimum 8 μV from the baseline EMG tone marks the start of period and should last at least 0.5 second to 10 seconds until the time when the EMG does not exceed 2 μV above resting. A minimum number of 4 such limb movements with a minimum period of 5 second and maximum until 90 seconds is required to score it as a limb movement. If the leg movements on both limbs are separated by less than 5 seconds, then they are considered a single event.

What Should Be Reported from an ECG Trace?

ECG recording from lead II can be used for screening various events. If the sampling rate is higher than 256 Hz, it is even better. As per current guidelines, 500 Hz is desired for this reason as it helps discern the events of higher frequencies better. Heart rate and its alterations can be reported for the night using the ECG trace. Sinus bradycardia less than 40 bpm, sinus tachycardia more than 90 bpm, asystole more than 3 seconds, with heart rate more than 100 bpm if the QRS duration is less than 120 ms, is scored as narrow complex tachycardia. It is scored as wide complex tachycardia if the QRS

duration is more than 120 ms for a consecutive 3 beats. Any evidence of atrial fibrillation, any other arrhythmia should be reported. Any sign of ischemia or infarction should be reported. At times these events may corroborate the technician notes during the night where it is recorded by the technician that the patient was uncomfortable, sweating, woke up with complaints of feeling not well, felt suffocated, needed to get a breath of fresh air and so woke up, and many other related complaints, and hence events should be also referred to the technician notes.

The ECG trace can be used along with pulse plethysmography trace to measure pulse transit time (PTT). PTT can be used to measure blood pressure indirectly.

Traces from the nasal cannula and oronasal cannula monitor pressure and are best to pick up hypopnea, while the oronasal thermistor indicates apnea by measuring the flow. Hypopnea is a more than 30% drop in peak signal as compared to pre-event baseline in the cannula trace. Duration should be more than 10 seconds. This reduced excursion may be associated with an arousal. Apnea is a sudden cessation of breath for more than 10 seconds as seen on the thermistor trace.

EMG trace at the chin can be used for bruxism, and limb leads may give a clue for REM behavior disorder. Arousal may lead to increased EMG tone in either of the traces.

Reporting of the Sleep Study

The patient profile should include, the vitals including age, weight, height, and BMI, symptoms in detail, and any questionnaires or other sleep workup like sleep diary results. The type of polysomnography should be indicated, along with the type of sensors used. Also list the following details:

- Lights off time
- Lights on time
- Total time in bed (TIB): The total duration of time from lights off to lights on
- Total sleep time (TST): The total duration of time while asleep in TIB
- Sleep onset latency (SOL): The duration of the onset of the first epoch of sleep from lights off (Average normal SOL ranges from 10 to 20 minutes.)

- Stage REM latency: The duration of the onset of the first epoch of REM from lights off
- Wake after sleep onset (WASO): Wake after sleep onset, calculated by subtracting the duration of SOL and TST from the TIB
- Sleep efficiency %: Calculated as a percentage of TST of TIB, normally more than 90%
- Duration of each stage—N1, N2, N3, REM, and wake: The duration of each stage in the entire TIB
- Stage as % of TST—N1%, N2%, N3%, REM%: The duration of each stage divided by the total sleep time as a percentage (N1% is about 5–10% of TST, N2 is 40–50% of TST, N3 is 20–25% of TST, and REM is 20–25% of TST approximately.)
- Average heart rate, minimum and maximum heart rate during the recording time while asleep and awake
- Scoring of events, done as per recommended guidelines and reported
- Arousal index
- Periodic limb movements index and its arousal index
- Respiratory-related arousals, arousal because of arrhythmia, desaturations
- Apnea hypopnea index, evidence of Bruxism, seizures, abnormal behavior and any cardiac event
- Summary of the notes of the sleep technician that may be related clinically
- Notes of the sleep lab in charge
- Summary of the case, indication of the polysomnography and suspicion of disorder, if any
- Suggested further investigations

The report should be signed, and the details of the lab, the contact number of the lab, the names of both who did the study and who signed the report should be legible and clear.

CONCLUSION

A good acquisition of data and grasp of the knowledge of the changes during sleep and of scoring sleep are the most important requirements for the study. A trained technician and a relatively noise-free room with a comfortable bed and bedding makes this type of study the gold standard. Though it is cost-intensive due to infrastructural, personnel, and equipment requirements, but, in complicated cases, it can clinch the diagnosis for better management and clinical outcomes.

SUGGESTED READING

1. Caples SM, Anderson WM, Calero K, Howell M, Hashmi SD. Use of polysomnography and home sleep apnea tests for the longitudinal management of obstructive sleep apnea in adults: an American Academy of Sleep Medicine clinical guidance statement. *J Clin Sleep Med.* 2021;17(6):1287–1293.
2. Aurora RN, Lamm CI, Zak RS, Kristo DA, Bista SR, Rowley JA, Casey KR. Practice parameters for the nonrespiratory indications for polysomnography and multiple sleep latency testing for children. *SLEEP.* 2012;35(11):1467–1473.
3. Aurora RN, Zak RS, Karippot A, Lamm CI, Morgenthaler TI, Auerbach SH, Bista SR, Casey KR, Chowdhuri S, Kristo DA, Ramar K. Practice parameters for the respiratory indications for polysomnography in children. *SLEEP.* 2011;34(3):379–388.
4. American Academy of Sleep Medicine. *International Classification of Sleep Disorders.* 3rd ed. Darien, IL: American Academy of Sleep Medicine; 2014.
5. AASM Manual for the Scoring of Sleep and Associated Events, Version 2.6.

21

Polysomnography II: Sample Reports with Explanation of Various Terminologies

DEEPAK SHRIVASTAVA

REVIEW OF SLEEP HYGIENE

Sleep hygiene is a practice of multiple behavior changes that lead to better-quality sleep. Good-quality sleep hygiene is important before scheduling a sleep study or for treating any sleep disorder. Sleep hygiene is one of the most important interventions that works on the basic physiologic principles and resets the sleep parameters to its natural form. Patient use of caffeine, and different forms should be discussed, and education provided. Significant marijuana smoking as well as other nicotine products should not be used close to bedtime. Routine exercise has significant value in regulating sleep. Maintenance of a comfortable bed and pillow, bedroom temperature and lighting, as well as a sleep-conducive ambience in the bedroom are important in accomplishing restorative sleep. The patient's inability to sleep sometimes stems from other coexistent insomnia or mostly generalized anxiety disorder (GAD) or situational anxiety. Multiple resources are available for intervention both with pharmaceutical and nonpharmaceutical approaches. Both medical and mental conditions tend to affect sleep negatively. The control of the comorbid conditions is important especially when it relates to chronic pain, gastrointestinal disturbance, and similar uncomfortable conditions. Review of patient medications, including prescription and over the counter, as well as herbal products, is important as nearly all the medications affect sleep negatively or positively. Many medications suppress REM sleep or non-REM sleep. Withdrawal from this medication can bring about a rebound of the suppressed sleep stage.

DOI: 10.1201/9781003093381-24

ORGANIZATION OF A SLEEP STUDY REPORT

After the overnight polysomnography, multiple parameters are recorded, and data are collected. As previously mentioned, these parameters record an electroencephalogram, electrooculogram, electromyogram, and electrocardiogram, as well as monitoring the airflow, chest movement abdominal movement, leg movements, and snoring oxygen saturation. The data are organized into different sections for reporting purposes. The sections include the patient identification and the demographic data, technical details regarding the process that was used in the setting of the sleep study with the methodology and review of monitored parameters. A summary of the patient's complaint, historical findings, and physical examination findings are recorded in the following section. This information is critical and applies the results of the sleep study to the patient's chief complaint, as well as the effect of the patient's comorbid conditions and medications on the sleep architecture as recorded. The next section records the cardiac activity and findings during sleep and respiratory events including apneas, hypopneas, respiratory-effort-related arousals, oxygen desaturation, and apnea hypopnea index.

Another section of the report is dedicated to the movement-related sleep disorders and records the periodic limb movements of sleep. After review of the findings as mentioned previously, an interpretive statement is made by the physician who reviewed the raw data and the compilation of findings in the sleep study report.

TERMINOLOGY REVIEW

The section that reports sleep architecture includes total recording time (TRT), time in bed (TIB), and total sleep time (TST).

TRT is the time that represents how long the recording equipment was activated while the patient was in bed.

TIB is important in establishing how long the subject was indeed trying to fall asleep. If the patient does not spend time in bed, then the total sleep time is going to be low and will cause symptoms consistent with insufficient sleep syndrome.

Sleep latency is the time from lights out to sleep onset. The upper end of sleep latency is considered to be 30 minutes. Long sleep latency is seen in patients with insomnia and other similar disorders. On the other hand, short sleep latency can be seen in patients who have been sleep deprived or who have taken certain medications with hypnotic effects. Special attention must be paid to the patient's habitual sleep time and wake time to adjust the lights out and lights on times during sleep study.

TST is the total sleep time that is scored from sleep onset to final awakening. The durations of awakenings in between are deducted from total sleep time. Total sleep time certainly provides significant information regarding the amount of sleep a patient is able to get.

- Short total sleep time can be seen in patients with insomnia, comorbid medical conditions, chronic pain, and sometimes medications or substance use.
- Long total sleep time can be seen in patients who are recovering from sleep deprivation or who have medical conditions affecting sleep. Medications and substance use can also increase total sleep time.

Sleep efficiency is the percentage of total time in bed compared to actual sleep recorded. Sleep efficiency is a good overall reflection of the quality of sleep.

- Low sleep efficiency can result from multiple factors that include long sleep latency and early morning awakenings with long sleep onset time.
- High sleep efficiency is associated with recovery sleep and the effect of the medications.

Wake after sleep onset (WASO) refers to the wakeful time during the sleep, between the sleep onset and sleep offset. This time is calculated by adding all the episodes of awakening during the night. WASO reflects sleep fragmentation and indicates nonrestorative sleep.

Wake time after sleep onset (WASO) reflects the early morning awakening generally seen in patients with depression. This can also be seen naturally in older age in the elderly with no difficulty in falling asleep but they wake up early after a short sleep.

REM latency is the time from sleep onset to the first episode of the REM sleep. It is affected by multiple factors, including the effect of the medications or withdrawal.

- Short REM latency can be seen in withdrawal from TCA antidepressant medications, MAO inhibitors, barbiturates, alcohol, and amphetamines. Many medical conditions like narcolepsy, sleep apnea, and depression also contribute to short REM latency.
- Long REM latency occurs when REM-suppressing medications are used; for example, TCA, intermittent amphetamine, alcohol, and barbiturates are some representative drugs.

SLEEP STAGES

This section of the polysomnography reports the percentage of area sleep stages. In general, stage N1 is approximately 5% of the total sleep time, stage N2 is 50%, stage N3 is 20%, and stage REM is 25% of the total sleep time.

Non-rapid Eye Movement (Non-REM) Sleep

Stage N1 sleep transitions from wakefulness to sleep and is a state of drowsiness. An increased quantity and percentage of N1 sleep reflect sleep fragmentation. It can be caused by the frequent arousals throughout the night. Clinical examples include periodic limb movements of sleep and obstructive sleep apnea.

Stage N2 sleep is the most prevalent sleep stage. It takes approximately 50% of the total sleep time. Increased N2 sleep is seen with age and medication effect. Decreased N2 sleep is a result of sleep fragmentation, increasing other stages of sleep like REM or stage N3. N2 sleep is also decreased in obstructive sleep apnea patients.

Stage N3 sleep is known by different names, including delta sleep or slow wave sleep. A high amount of N3 sleep is seen in the first half of the night. Increased N3 sleep is noted in rebound sleep after sleep deprivation or after the initiation of positive airway pressure therapy in sleep disordered breathing patients. Decreased N3 sleep is seen with effective medications, especially benzodiazepines, barbiturates, and TCAs.

RAPID EYE MOVEMENT (REM) SLEEP

REM sleep constitutes approximately 25% of the total sleep time. REM sleep generally dominates the second half of the night. REM sleep alternates with non-REM sleep in cycles of 80–110 minutes. A total of 4–5 cycles can be completed during 1 night of sleep. As the night progresses, the length of the REM sleep continues to gradually increase with the longest REM in the early morning hours.

An increase in REM sleep was noted in recovery sleep after sleep deprivation and withdrawal from REM-suppressing medications.

A decrease in REM sleep occurs with the effect of medications like barbiturates, TCAs, MAO inhibitors, and anticholinergic medications and after meals.

REVIEW OF RESPIRATORY EVENTS

Respiratory events are reported in a separate section. This is one of the most important sections of the report as the diagnosis of sleep disordered breathing is based on the findings of the recorded events calculated per hour of sleep. The following five events are reported:

Obstructive apnea: Cessation of airflow from the nose and mouth lasting 10 seconds or longer that may or may not have accompanying SA02 desaturation

Central apnea: Cessation of airflow from the nose and mouth and absence of diaphragmatic and abdominal efforts lasting 10 seconds or longer; may or may not have accompanying SA02 desaturation

Mixed apnea: Cessation of airflow from the nose and mouth, beginning with the absence of diaphragmatic and abdominal efforts lasting 10 seconds or longer; may or may not have accompanying SA02 desaturation

Hypopnea: A decrease in airflow from the nose and mouth and a decrease in amplitude of diaphragmatic and abdominal efforts lasting 10 seconds or longer, followed by an arousal that must be associated with 02 desaturation equal to or greater than 3%

Respiratory-effort-related arousal (RERA): Previously called upper airway resistance syndrome, the progressively increased effort to breathe in the setting of declining flow, eventually ending in cortical arousal and awakening of the patient (No oxygen desaturation is noted.)

The **apnea-hypopnea index (AHI)** is the sum of total apneas and hypopneas noted over the total sleep time. The apnea hypopnea index is arguably the most important parameter documented in the sleep study report. The index allows the provider to assess the risk of potential complications related to sleep disordered breathing (obstructive sleep apnea). Treatment decisions are based on the apnea-hypopnea index, which serves as a measure of the efficacy of the applied treatment.

The apnea hypopnea index is:

- Normal if it is less than 5.
- Mild from 5 to 14 events per hour.
- Moderate from 15 to 30 events per hour.
- Severe over 30 events per hour.

The **respiratory distress index (RDI)** is the sum of total apneas, hypopneas, and respiratory-effort-related arousals.

REVIEW OF PERIODIC LIMB MOVEMENTS

Periodic limb movements are repetitive movements that frequently involve flexion of the toes, ankle, knee, and hip. Due to these movements, some patients report difficulty falling asleep or sleep maintenance insomnia. These movements can impact daytime functioning and can cause fatigue and daytime sleepiness.

They are generally divided into:

- Limb movements in sleep (PLMS) frequently noted when the limb activity is monitored by EMG during sleep.
- Periodic limb movement disorder (PLMD) is documented when the periodic limb movement of sleep is associated with daytime or nighttime symptoms.

If PLMs are found to be part of another sleep disorder like restless leg syndrome (RLS), then the underlying primary sleep disorder should be treated.

Periodic limb movements index in wake and sleep are:

- Normal PLMI < 15 adults.
- Abnormal PLMI > 15 in adults.

The movements occur during REM (loss of atonia).

AROUSAL EVENTS

The total number of arousals and awakenings is reported as a frequency per hour of sleep and is referred to as an index. Even with a mild arousal index, obviously sleep is interrupted and will cause daytime symptoms of tiredness and fatigue.

$$\text{Arousal index} = \text{Total number of arousals per hour of sleep}$$

or

$$\text{Number of arousals} \times \text{PLMS/TST in minutes}$$

PARASOMNIA VIDEO RECORDING

Video recordings are important in capturing the details of patient behavior, activity, and abnormal movements; video complements the waveform recordings and makes the interpretations more accurate. Video and audio features are important both in adults and in pediatric sleep studies. Video recording truly enhances the quality of the sleep study and allows identification of the disorders that may not be obvious from the waveform analysis:

- Sleepwalking, sleep talking
- Bruxism ≥2 events with audible sound and polysomnographic evidence
- REM sleep behavior disorder (RBD) (no consensus concerning the number of REM epochs without atonia)

CARDIAC EVENTS DURING SLEEP

Cardiac monitoring documents normal electrical activity of the heart and cardiac arrhythmias in different sleep stages. Data from a solitary EEG lead are used to identify cardiac rhythm disturbances and other abnormalities.

- **Sinus tachycardia:** A sustained sinus heart rate >90 beats/minute for adults
- **Bradycardia:** A sustained heart rate <40/minute for age 6 years–adults
- **Asystole:** Cardiac pauses >3 seconds for ages 6 years–adult
- **Wide complex tachycardia:** A minimum of 3 consecutive beats at a rate >100/minute with QRS duration ≥120 ms
- **Narrow complex tachycardia:** A minimum of 3 consecutive beats at a rate ≥100/min with QRS duration < 120 ms

The technologist should also add any significant medical or sleep-related information discovered during patient assessment, while being tested, or before discharge: comments on sleep architecture, behavioral observations, myoclonus/limb movements, respiratory characteristics including respiratory events and desaturations, initiation of PAP, if applicable, and heart rate/ECG observations.

HYPNOGRAM

A hypnogram is a composite graphic display of the overnight sleep-wake stages, respiratory events, and other recorded parameters in the polysomnogram. The hypnogram gives a bird's-eye view on a single page, where events can be correlated to the activity occurring at the same time in different channels. Sleep structure can be easily characterized by review of the hypnogram:

- Panoramic graphic view
- Excellent account of sleep stages
- Apnea and hypopnea events, oxygen saturation, arousals, chest and abdominal movements, and body position, all in real time
- If CPAP is used, visualization of the effect of positive pressure on sleep and airflow parameters
- An overall excellent clinical impression

PRACTICE IMPLICATIONS

The report of the sleep study is an excellent document not only that provides information regarding the confirmation of the clinical diagnosis as it relates to the patient's chief complaint but that has comprehensive details regarding the different stages of sleep on the timeline of 6–8 hours of total sleep time. These parameters and observations help in clinical decision making and recommendations regarding better-quality sleep. Each parameter derived from the collected data has a significant impact on the general information and lifestyle changes. A focused recommendation can be made regarding changes to be made in sleep time, exercise, and substance use. It also shows the impact of different medical and psychiatric conditions as well as the medication effect on the overall quality of the sleep. Appropriate adjustments can be made in the management of these disorders or medications.

If the sleep study includes CPAP titration, then further recommendations can be made regarding the pressure to be used and the type of the mask interface, humidity settings, as well as the ramp function settings.

Review of the sleep study further emphasizes patient follow-up on a regular basis in order to troubleshoot any improvement-related problems and to assess the efficacy of the CPAP therapy. Sometimes underlying disorders surface once the obstructive sleep apnea is treated. These visits provide an opportunity to discover other disorders that were not evident due to the presence of sleep disordered breathing.

SUGGESTED READING

1. Pressman MR. *Primer of Polysomnogram Interpretation*. Boston: Butterworth Heinemann; 2002 [Google Scholar].
2. Shrivastava D, Jung S, Saadat M, Sirohi R, Crewson K. How to interpret the results of a sleep study. *J Community Hosp Intern Med Perspect.* 2014;4(5):24983. http://doi.org/10.3402/jchimp.v4.24983.
3. Prabhudesai P, Patankar M, Vardhan A. Sleep study interpretation in obstructive sleep apnea. *Int J Head Neck Surg.* 2019;10(2):42–46.
4. AASM Manual for the Scoring of Sleep and Associated Events, Version 2.6.

PART 4

What Should I Do Now? (Management)

22

Sleep Hygiene Principles and Nonpharmacological Interventions including Light Therapy

KARUNA DATTA

INTRODUCTION

The nonpharmacological approach to a sleep problem may be used to avoid development of a sleep disorder in cases where the sleep problem is still a symptom and not a disorder. It can be used as an adjunct in the overall management of sleep disorders.

Though the nonpharmacological approach is often referred to for insomnia, it may also be applied to lifestyle modifications for weight loss, especially for obstructive sleep apnea, cognitive behavioral therapy (CBT), and for disorders other than insomnia, e.g., depression, anxiety etc. Positive airway pressure and oral appliance therapy for the management of obstructive sleep apnea are discussed in detail in Chapters 25 and 26. Similarly, a behavioral approach is found to be effective for children with bed wetting problems and night waking, but that is beyond the scope of this chapter.

This chapter emphasizes on the nonpharmacological approach in adults for chronic insomnia, which includes principles of sleep hygiene, CBT for insomnia (CBTI), complementary and alternative therapy, and the use of light as a therapeutic option for sleep disorders.

COGNITIVE, PSYCHOLOGICAL, AND BEHAVIORAL TREATMENT

As per AASM guidelines, multicomponent CBTI is strongly recommended for treatment of chronic insomnia patients. It usually takes 4–8 sessions, and the effect starts to appear gradually and steadily.

CBT suitability to the patient should be judged by both the referring primary care physician and the therapist. CBTI includes sleep restriction, stimulus control therapy, relaxation-based interventions, cognitive strategies, and sleep hygiene education. For insomnia, it is aimed at the pathophysiology of insomnia explained by Spielman's 3P model: precipitating, predisposing, and perpetuating factors. These factors can be specifically identified in the patient with regular interviews and noted. Predispositions added with perpetuating

DOI: 10.1201/9781003093381-26

factors precipitate conditions to prolong the insomnia. Once the factors are clear, a directed approach toward developing strategies to mitigate them can be developed.

Behavioral therapy is comprised of sleep hygiene, sleep restriction, stimulus control, and relaxation training. Cognitive strategy aims at restructuring cognitive beliefs that hamper sleep. This multicomponent therapy using cognitive and behavioral therapy comprises CBTI.

The idea of CBTI is not to change personality traits but insight-oriented psychotherapy with respect to the predisposing and perpetuating factors. CBTI is based on the premise of maladaptive cognitions that, according to Beck's theory, include general beliefs about the world, the self, and the future, giving rise to specific and automatic thoughts in particular situations that, when targeted with therapeutic strategies, lead to changes in emotional distress and behaviors. Patients motivated to work on their maladaptive beliefs perform better. Specific problem areas, once identified, help the therapist to formulate specific targeted goals for therapy. The therapy is gradual and slow to show improvement, and hence observing patience on the part of the patient and therapist is the key to successful outcomes.

Multicomponent CBTI is comprised of sleep hygiene, sleep education, sleep restriction, stimulus control, and relaxation therapy.

SLEEP RESTRICTION

In this component of multicomponent CBTI, the individual is instructed to restrict the time in bed. This is done to improve sleep efficiency, which is the time slept divided by the time in bed as a percentage. If the sleep efficiency is lesser than 85%, sleep restriction can reduce the time in bed, hence increasing the sleep efficiency percentage. The amount of time in bed should not be reduced to less than 6 hours in any case. Such sleep restriction can cause sleep deprivation and, in some patients, may cause daytime fatigue, sleepiness during daytime, irritability, and attention problems due to lack of sleep. Hence the clinician should avoid further sleep restriction in patients complaining of the side effects just mentioned due to sleep deprivation effects. It is contraindicated in heavy-duty machine operators, patients with history of mania or hypomania, and cases predisposed to or suffering from seizure disorders.

STIMULUS CONTROL

The bed or bedroom is associated with sleep or sexual activity. The individual is asked to follow this strictly such that the stimulus of bed or being in the bedroom becomes associated with sleeping. If the patient is not able to sleep for 15–20 minutes after lying in bed to sleep, the individual is advised to get out of bed and return when sleepy. A fixed wake-up time is advised to be followed.

RELAXATION THERAPY

Relaxation therapy is an important component of CBTI. It aims to reduce sleep onset or wake after sleep onset. Progressive muscular relaxation is frequently used. Appropriate training for the individual should be imparted by the therapist to instill confidence in the patient and to ensure compliance.

SLEEP HYGIENE

Sleep hygiene alone as a single component is not recommended by the AASM for treatment of chronic insomnia in adults. Sleep hygiene principles are habits that improve sleep. They can be explained in two ways. First is a didactic method, in which all the principles are explained to the individual. Second, the points that need to be dealt with due to the individual's complaining of the inability to sleep or due to a problem are addressed after a brief interview analyzing the individual's habits. The principles of sleep hygiene primarily involve the habit of making a consistent routine with a set bedtime and wake time for both weekdays and weekends. It includes indulging in relaxing activities and avoiding stimulants before sleep. Stimulants like smoking before bedtime are best avoided. Alcohol is often misused to help in falling asleep. Though the patient goes off to sleep after becoming drunk, the effect of alcohol is actually deleterious to sleep. It affects the maintenance of sleep and causes frequent awakenings and an unrefreshed sleep. It is recommended to avoid alcohol at bedtime. In the case of increased presleep arousal, reserve caffeine for the morning hours. A relaxed schedule at bedtime, and the avoidance of bright light exposure before sleep helps.

Though these are general tips for improving sleep in a healthy population, in sleep disorders it becomes an important part of the nonpharmacological approach to the patient management strategy.

Some points for patients:

- Keep a consistent bedtime and wakeup time. The total time in bed should be at least 7–8 hours; adequate opportunity to sleep should be provided by the patient for sleep. Having a consistent bedtime and wakeup time both on weekdays and weekends is crucial to avoid sleep deprivation. Unless the patient needs to entrain to a new timing, which should be planned as per the disorder under consultation, this consistent schedule should be followed.
- Avoid studying in bed and only use bed for sleep and sex.
- Unwind before sleep time. Indulge in relaxing activities and avoid stimulants before bedtime. Alcohol consumption before bedtime is known to deteriorate sleep quality. After alcohol, the patient may sleep easily and so is even used to go to sleep in cases of sleep onset insomnia, but alcohol makes the patient keep on waking up during the night and impairs the sleep quality. Smoking before sleep time should be best avoided due to the stimulant action on the body. Caffeine should be restricted from the afternoon onwards, if one is sensitive and sleep onset is affected. Preferably no caffeine within 4–5 hours of bedtime is a good habit to follow even if there is no sleep problem.
- A healthy exercise schedule during the morning hours helps sleep. The time of exercise should be preferably morning and best avoided just before sleep time. The intensity of the exercise should be mild to moderate and never severe, especially if done during evening. Severe exercise can delay sleep in some insomnia patients, but a moderate to vigorous exercise schedule may be beneficial for OSA patients. The vigorous exercise protocol, however, should be done only with the consultation of the physician and under supervision to avoid deleterious effects on the heart. Mild to moderate exercise done in the morning hours is found to advance sleep that evening. Patients with circadian rhythm disorder should be watched for their requirements, their biological day and night, and prescribed exercise as a lifestyle intervention.
- Food habits are important. Do not have very heavy meals before sleep time. Avoid lots of fluids just before sleep time. Spicy foods cause trouble at night by causing reflux, and foods rich in tyramine (e.g., cheese, bacon, etc.) cause problem sleeping and hence are best avoided. Warm milk is known to induce sleep due to the high tryptophan in it, and it relaxes the individual. A word of caution for patients with lactose intolerance and for those who cannot tolerate fluids: avoid milk near sleep time.
- Avoid long afternoon naps. A nap should not be more than 20–40 minutes. Frequent naps during the daytime are best avoided in the healthy population. In cases of advanced sleep-wake disorders, naps may be beneficial to prescribe for these patients. Naps in these patients can help them perform better during the latter part of the day, especially if they are elderly. The exact time of the nap needs consultation.

Sleep education can be done using a 2-week sleep diary of the individual. This makes the interaction more individualized.

Multicomponent CBTI is strongly recommended for the treatment of chronic insomnia in adults. When the initial side effects are seen to be due to sleep restriction, a gradual change in habits and cognitive restructuring has been found to show a higher benefit-to-harm ratio. However, in cases of comorbid medical or psychiatric conditions, the benefit-to-harm ratio must be considered before or during CBTI, and the therapist should be vigilant about the side effects. Cases where sleep restriction is to be avoided or sleep deprivation effects are not desired, clinician must keep a note of the benefit-to-harm ratio before advising CBTI.

Multicomponent brief therapy for insomnia includes reduced CBT sessions, which may be only 1–4 in number, along with sleep restriction, stimulus control, and relaxation therapies. As per AASM guidelines, multicomponent brief therapies may be used as therapy, though multicomponent CBTI is strongly recommended. In cases where patients are unable to come for 4–8 sessions of CBTI or cannot afford them, behavioral therapy may be taken. As with CBTI, the side effects due to sleep deprivation should be looked for, and patients contraindicated for sleep restriction should not be administered a sleep restriction component.

Brief behavioral treatment of insomnia alone has a rapid effect but is not sustained and hence cognitive therapy, which is slower but sustainable, should be added. It is proposed that the treatment be more individualized.

Though CBTI remains the first line of therapy for insomnia, it is often underutilized primarily due to two main factors: patient-centered and system-based issues.

Patient-centered Reasons

- Lack of time for 4–8 sessions
- Cost involved
- Difficulty in maintaining the prescribed sleep-wake regimes
- Stigma of psychotherapy
- Laziness on the part of a patient who just wants a simple pill to "cure" insomnia rather than working on behavioral changes

System-based Issues

- Lack of provider awareness regarding CBTI effectiveness
- Limits on the patient's visit length
- Insurance coverage difficulties or difficulties in payments
- Limited availability of CBTI-trained specialists

These problems can be overcome by increasing awareness among patients, increased training, and hence increased availability of trained CBTI therapists, by trying an online mode of providing CBTI, or by a combination using hybrid sessions of face-to-face offline and online sessions both, etc.

Also, there is a need to develop other management options. Mindfulness meditation has been tried as a form of relaxation training along with CBT in insomnia patients. AASM guidelines suggest that clinicians use sleep restriction, stimulus control, or relaxation therapy as a single component therapy for chronic insomnia in adults as conditional implying that the "clinician uses clinical knowledge and experience, and to strongly consider the patient's values and preferences to determine the best course of action."

COMPLEMENTARY AND ALTERNATE MEDICINE

The U.S. National Institutes of Health has classified yoga as a holistic approach to health, and it is considered a form of Complementary and Alternative Medicine. With this has emerged a new concept of "therapeutic yoga." Studies have used yoga nidra, acupuncture, Tai Chih Chi, hypnosis, and mindfulness meditation for the treatment of insomnia.

Efforts have been made to use these options in patients. A need to develop a therapeutic model for the use of yoga or meditation is essential. To make it a standardized practice, guidelines as to how to use the practice as a therapeutic option, the patients for whom the practice is contraindicated, checkpoints to keep in mind while the patient is doing the practice, and what side effects may be anticipated, if any, should be explained to the patient and the instructor.

Models using mindfulness meditation and yoga nidra have been tried in chronic insomnia patients.

Using a complementary or alternate medicine approach in insomnia patients, like any other method, requires constant supervision by the treating physician. Care should be taken to ensure that the patient takes up the yoga postures after consultation, e.g., forward bending postures are contraindicated for gastroesophageal reflux cases, and focused meditation is best avoided by patients having anxiety. Patients with psychiatric comorbidity should do meditation or yoga nidra only after consultation with a psychiatrist.

Lifestyle interventions based on principles for sleep disorders can include an exercise prescription and diet charts. A thought record can be done before going to bed to avoid carrying problems to bed before going to sleep. Exercises can be done specially for toning the neck muscles, facial muscles, and belly to help in obstructive sleep apnea. A well-timed exercise, exposure to sunlight or bright light, and maintaining social cues to promote good sleep can help in circadian rhythm disorders and might help insomniacs.

LIGHT AS A THERAPEUTIC OPTION

The effect of light on circadian rhythm varies with the timing at which it is given. It has been found that if bright light is given before the body core temperature is minimum (CBT_{min}), it delays the sleep-wake cycle and that, if it is given after the CBT_{min}, it advances the sleep cycle. So, in a normal sleep-wake cycle that is coordinated with light and dark phases, bright light exposure in the evening delays sleep and in the morning causes advancement in sleep at night. For artificial means of therapy, then, it is important to determine CBT_{min}. The most sensitive time for the light phase response curve is usually 2–3 hours before and after CBT_{min}. Hence the light exposure should be timed according to the CBT_{min}.

Indications

Light therapy is recommended by AASM for adults with advanced sleep-wake phase syndrome vs. no treatment and for elderly and dementia cases of irregular sleep-wake rhythm disorder. However, its use with melatonin is not recommended for elderly with dementia cases. Light therapy is also recommended for jet lag disorder and in shift work disorder patients.

Delivery of light can be done from a natural source or by artificial means. The advantage of a natural source is the relative ease and the low cost, but the disadvantage—or rather the need for the artificial means of delivery of light—is always the inaccessibility of the natural source at the time required. The artificial source can be given to the patient during nighttime too.

Delivery of light by artificial source involves the following requirements:

- The light should be oriented in such a way that it is presented to the individual from above, since the lower part of the retina has an enhanced effect on suppression of melatonin.
- Choosing the spectrum of light, with filters if required, the output intensity, the size of source, and the positioning of the irradiating surface needs to be decided. Glare should be reduced, and heat emission should not be uncomfortable. The portability of the equipment, if required by the patient, determines the choice of the equipment.
- Artificial sources of light can be:
  - A light box of a standard size of 2×4 feet kept on a table 3 feet away from the user.
  - Fluorescent lamps or lights. For fluorescent lamps, the ballast frequency should be as per the requirement.
- The light-generating device should be validated and conform to the standards for therapeutics.
- The adverse effects of bright light therapy should always be kept in mind. Incandescent lamps should never be used for light therapy as their illumination is harmful to the retinal pigment epithelium. Very small devices used for light therapy also are not advisable as a small change in head position can affect the amount of light reaching the retina and thus change the chronobiotic effect. Broad field illumination is preferred and can even be given while the sleeper is sleeping as a dawn stimulation. Naturalistic dawn can be created with 250 lux of light intensity.
- Light therapy can be a problem in cases with a history of photosensitive medications; examples are drugs like phenothiazines, antimalarials, psoralen, etc. Retinopathy is an absolute contraindication for bright light therapy. Also, it may not be acceptable for patients with eye diseases and for some who experience light-therapy-related headaches. Constant supervision should be done of patients, and consultation of ophthalmologists or dermatologists may be considered before starting it and also during the treatment.

There is an individual susceptibility to the effect of light on melatonin suppression, and hence individualized treatment under supervision is always recommended. Natural lighting is preferred for therapy. Exposure to light in the morning hours and avoidance to bright light before sleeping is one of the most inexpensive yet effective methods of light therapy.

A combination therapy using behavioral treatment using natural light exposure in the morning, following sleep hygiene principles, and postawakening light therapy has been found to show some therapeutic evidence, though weak for adults and children suffering from delayed sleep phase syndrome. For the use of light therapy in various circadian rhythm disorders, see Chapter 13.

SUGGESTED READING

1. Edinger JD, Arnedt JT, Bertisch SM, et al. Behavioral and psychological treatments for chronic insomnia disorder in adults: an American Academy of Sleep Medicine clinical practice guideline. *J Clin Sleep Med.* 2021;17(2):255–262. https://doi.org/10.5664/jcsm.8986

2. Datta K, Tripathi M, Mallick HN. *Yoga Nidra*: an innovative approach for management of chronic insomnia: a case report. *Sleep Sci Pract*. 2017;1:7. https://doi.org/10.1186/s41606-017-0009-4

3. Ong J, Sholtes D. A mindfulness-based approach to the treatment of insomnia. *J Clin Psychol*. 2010;66(11):1175–1184. http://doi.org/10.1002/jclp.20736.

4. Eastman CI, Burgess HJ. How to travel the world without jet lag. *Sleep Med Clin*. 2009;4(2):241–255. http://doi.org/10.1016/j.jsmc.2009.02.006.

5. Datta K, Tripathi M, Mallick HN. *Yoga Nidra*: an innovative approach for management of chronic insomnia: a case report. *Sleep Sci Pract*. 2017;1:7. https://doi.org/10.1186/s41606-017-0009-4.

23

Identifying the Need for Counselling

KARUNA DATTA

INTRODUCTION

A need to know when to send an individual for counselling becomes practically important for sleep problems for the simple reason of preventing further deterioration of the problem. Patients often go unnoticed because their telltale signs are missed during outpatient consultations by physicians who are not looking for them. This relative lack of proactiveness increases the patient burden on society. The requirement of counselling needs to be picked up early so that it can be nipped in the bud, e.g., for college students or schoolchildren, a faint glimpse of a problem can be corrected faster and more permanently than when it is addressed after many years of simmering inside, probably erupting into a full-blown disease or disorder.

This chapter deals with a listing of certain red flags that a health practitioner or school or college counsellor shouldn't miss. Three case scenarios are laid out to focus the objectives more clearly.

Let's start the chapter with the first case scenario.

CASE SCENARIO 1

A 16-year-old class X student, Subhash, is commonly found quarrelling with his classmates. The teachers had found him often dozing or yawning in class. This was, however, a recent phenomenon. He was a good student and had been scoring reasonably well in high school, but recently his term results showed a dip in performance. He was being ticked off by teachers and teased by classmates. One of the experienced teachers saw this change in Subhash and spoke to him in an empathetic manner about his academics and school/home environment. It was learned that his relatives had come from the village 2 months back and were staying with them. He had to share the room where he used to study and sleep. Because of this there had been a change in his study schedule. He had to sleep at times when the lights were still on, share a bed with two snoring adults, and tend to their demands off and on. This had led to increased sleep deprivation and probably to his reduced work efficiency.

DOI: 10.1201/9781003093381-27

CASE SCENARIO 2

A 50-year-old entrepreneur, an old case of hypertension and diabetes on regular treatment, came to the OPD with complaints of not being able to sleep for the past 2–3 weeks once or twice a week after going to bed. His financial year closure was near, and he said that sometimes a thought might just come to him before sleeping, and it would keep him busy planning or thinking, which would compromise his sleep onset. Because of this, he would wake up late and feel unrefreshed, which further compromised his work and increased his worry. The doctor noticed that his blood pressure was also elevated despite being on two antihypertensives and one diuretic.

As a primary care physician, it is a rather common sight. Often, we don't think of anything to offer. Can we offer a counselling session?

WHAT IS COUNSELLING?

Counselling is a one-on-one method where a counsellor and the person seeking counselling, referred to as a counselee, interact in a nonthreatening, safe environment. "Safe" implies that this interaction happens because of mutual trust and faith developed between the counsellor and counselee. Therefore, it may take some time for the actual counselling session to be effective. The objective of the counselling session is to enable the counselee to identify the problem and seek acceptance and self-direction. The counselee finds the way to find solutions to his or her problems and determines methods in which to overcome them. Note that merely providing information and giving advice is not considered counselling.

COUNSELLOR–COUNSELEE INTERACTION

Mutual respect is vital for a successful interaction between counsellor and counselee. The counselee should be able to accept the counsellor. After the initial engagement, the counsellor allows the counselee to share the problem and fully express the emotional content. With active listening and open discussion, the counsellor can make the counselee aware of various factors causing the problem. Subsequently, through an effective problem solving and decision-making

technique, the counsellor empowers the counselee to select the most compatible solution to the problem. Subsequently, evaluation focuses on the effectiveness of the method adapted and suitable modifications, if any, for the achievement and maintenance of the desired goal.

While the counselee states the problem, the counsellor needs to:

- Make the counselee comfortable and able to converse freely.
- Have unconditional positive regard toward the counselee.
- Identify the problem(s) affecting the counselee with active listening and empathetic probing.
- Identify the resources, personal attributes, coping skills, and home/school environment that the counsellor brings to the counselee.
- Be able to clarify for the patient how certain issues are causing these problems and how they can be modified for a solution.
- Empower the counselee to come up with the most compatible solution from the various strategies discussed.
- Make short-term and long-term goals for follow-up.
- Entertain the flexibility to change strategy or modify goals on subsequent visits based on the outcome of earlier visits.

RED FLAGS WHEN A PERSON IS COMPLAINING OF SLEEP PROBLEMS

- Increased daytime sleepiness/yawning
- Inability to maintain focus on work as usual
- Undue fatigue/tiredness
- Undue irritability/mood swings
- Making mistakes/accidents at the workplace
- A recent dip in performance
- Excessive critical evaluation of self
- Unexplained fear/sadness/anxiety
- Any other daytime consequences due to the sleep problem

CASE SCENARIO 3 (COUNSELLING SESSION)

"I am not able to sleep properly." Robin looked tired, had dark circles beneath his eyes and horizontal furrows on his forehead.

"Have a seat. Are you comfortable? Tell me more about it," the counsellor said.

Robin: "I have been studying till late for my college exams. I go to bed at 12 midnight but am unable to sleep till 3 o'clock. Sometimes I toss and turn the entire night and feel I have been awake the entire night."

"Oh . . . I see. So please tell me in detail. What do you do when you don't get to sleep?" the counsellor quickly inquired.

Robin: "I keep thinking about my preparation, future or take my book and read till the time I start feeling asleep."

"Do you mean to say you are worried about your future? And your anxiety makes you lose your sleep?" asked the counsellor.

Robin: "Maybe, how would I know?"

"You tell me. Are you unduly worried about the exam? Do you get restless, jittery, anxious during daytime? Is your sleep disturbance greater when you are preoccupied or anxious? Tell me more about your life and routine," the counsellor said.

Robin: "Actually, I have been a good student and wanted to get admission in medicine. My parents could not afford my entrance fees at the time, so I joined another course and apart from my studies, I started taking home tuitions for schoolchildren to make ends meet. I thought it would be easy for me, but it is very tough. In fact, I felt very dejected the other day, when my school friends mentioned how they are taking extra courses, classes, and tuitions, and here I am, doing college, taking tuitions for children, and trying to compete with my classmates. Some of my school mates who are not that bright are faring better than me."

"It's nice to know," the counsellor responded, "that you are putting in so much effort to take another attempt at the course you so much desire. You have good grades, and you are intelligent; in what way are these courses different from your school examinations?" The counsellor was trying to understand.

Robin: "Quite different. These courses are very application based and require in-depth understanding of many concepts, and many of them were trick questions. Just merely covering the topic did not help much; rather I needed more time to get the answer than I had anticipated despite covering the entire curriculum."

"So, you mean to say that you were not prepared for it. What would make you better equipped?" the counsellor asked.

Robin: "Well, I think first I need to stop worrying about it and rather develop a strategy to get it over with successfully. I think I need to change my approach and practice more of the questions rather than the theory alone. Concentrate on increasing my speed and accuracy too. Do as many of them as I can. Devise some mnemonics to remember important repetitive concepts but tricky ones, which are difficult to remember."

"That's nice. Will you be able to give it a try now? Is it possible for you to do some practice questions? Can you purchase some preparation material?" added the counsellor.

Robin: "I will try. I think I might get some material from my seniors too. I can also study with some of my school friends. Sujoy had offered. I think I can try that out. My semester exams finish in a week's time and after that I can concentrate on these."

"Great. So, let's try this out. By worrying about what will happen next week, you are unable to focus now. I believe this strategy might help you," added the counsellor.

Robin: "Yes sure. You are right, I was probably stressed out. I think I will get good sleep today."

"See, stress, and sleep are quite interrelated. While stress might affect your sleep, sleep disturbance can give you physical and emotional distress. If we do not follow good sleep hygiene, it affects our body adversely, and leads to stress, anxiety, or even mental illness. Whereas good sleep habits may eliminate such possibilities in the future as well. There are strategies that improve both sleep as well as anxiety. Would you like to know more?"

"Sure, that would be great . . ."

. . . And this is how the first counselling session of Robin went. We can appreciate the various steps brought out by the counsellor to make Robin comfortable and help him analyze his problem. Mutually, they developed a strategy, and Robin was receptive and involved in the planning throughout.

Subsequently, if Robin is not able to handle the situation regularly, he might need a revision of strategy or might need a consultation for more specific therapies like cognitive behavioral therapy. That will unfold in future sessions. Hence, for a counsellor, it is important to review and evaluate the condition for some time until the counselee finds the solution or develops the confidence to handle it further.

The need to take counselling should be identified by the health practitioner while attending to the medical condition, as in Case Scenario 2. Also, as in Scenarios 1 and 3, it is important for parents, teachers, and health attendants to identify the need for a counsellor in an otherwise seemingly normal person with subtle changes in behavior.

HOW IS COUNSELLING DIFFERENT FROM COGNITIVE BEHAVIORAL THERAPY (CBT)?

In CBT, the therapist aims at working together with the individual on changing behavior and restructuring cognitively, i.e., modifying the thinking patterns and beliefs of the individual that hamper health. Counselling, on the other hand, helps the individual to identify the problem and formulate strategies to help cope with the issues. Here the counsellor makes Robin understand himself enough to find his own solutions and hopes that Robin follows them. It is less directive than CBT.

WHEN CAN ONE REFER FOR COUNSELLING?

A timely counselling may ward off a brewing disorder/disease. Counselling may detect the problem at an early stage and may offer a solution through simple lifestyle modification. Counselling for sleep-related issues should be a problem-based intervention and not an illness-based intervention. Many factors in routine life events can cause sleep disturbances without causing an illness, and the remedy for that can be simple and effective, with sleep-related counselling.

Counselling may be done by any health care worker trained in the basics of counselling. Counselling may be provided by a doctor who is treating an individual for an associated problem, such as a case of hypertension or diabetes with an associated sleep disturbance. Also, a primary care physician might feel a need to refer for cognitive behavioral therapy but, due to a lack of availability of a trained counsellor in the vicinity, may ask the patient to go for counselling instead. Sometimes the patient needs "talk time" to vent about the problems and can find a solution as Robin did in our case. Hence identifying the need and referring to a counsellor may be the only thing required. Primary care physicians should use their clinical discretion, especially when there is lack of trained personnel for CBT or when it is not feasible for the patient to go to the therapist frequently because of time and money constraints. However, monitoring and regular follow-ups must be made by the physician, and the patient must not be left on his or her own after referral to the counsellor.

CONCLUSION

Counselling remains an important component of therapy, especially in patients suffering with sleep problems and sleep disorders. Identifying the need for counselling by parents, teachers, peers, employers, students, patients, doctors, therapists, psychologists, and others remains pivotal in identifying and accepting the issue so that an early measure may be planned and implemented. Evaluation of the planned strategy is also an important role of the counsellor, who can help refer the individual to the doctor or therapist or for further counselling sessions as the need may be.

ACKNOWLEDGMENT

The author acknowledges Dr. Jyoti Prakash, MD (Psy), MAMS, PDC Child (Psy), PGDM, PGDCA, WHO Fellow (Johns Hopkins), Professor, Department of Psychiatry, Armed Forces Medical College, Pune, Maharashtra, India for reviewing this manuscript and providing his valuable suggestions.

24

Pharmacological Agents Used in Various Sleep Disorders

DEEPAK SHRIVASTAVA

HYPNOTICS AND SEDATIVES

Multiple medications and substances have been used historically to induce sleep. In addition, the general pharmaceutical population has used alcohol and other substances easily available to fall asleep. Benzodiazepines and barbiturates, just like alcohol, modulate the GABA receptors and are commonly used medications to treat insomnia. Although not frequently used, chloral hydrate and all compounds are still used for sleep addiction.

BENZODIAZEPINE RECEPTOR AGONIST DRUGS (BZRA)

BZRAs are common drugs used for the treatment of insomnia. There are old GABA receptor modulators like temazepam, flurazepam, and estazolam. Then the newer BZRAs with a much different chemical structure interact with GABA receptors, namely zolpidem, zaleplon, eszopiclone, and quazepam. Benzodiazepines have better safety profiles compared to drugs like barbiturates, which can cause respiratory depression, sedation, a coma-like state, or even death. Zolpidem is considered a safer medication to induce more physiologic sleep. It has only few withdrawal symptoms and is less likely to cause drug tolerance.

Effects on Sleep

Benzodiazepine receptor antagonists can cause sedation, relieve anxiety, induce muscle relaxation, decrease sleep onset time, and cause amnesia. From the sleep architecture point of view, a decrease in initial sleep latency and an increase in total sleep time are the most effective advantages of losing these drugs. They decrease the stage N1 sleep and slow wave N3 sleep. The N2 sleep amount is increased. These agents increase REM sleep latency and decrease total REM sleep time. Zolpidem, zaleplon, and eszopiclone do not have any effect on N3 slow wave sleep. Benzodiazepine receptor antagonist drugs are classified according to their timing and duration of effect into short-acting, intermediate-acting, and long-acting medications.

Triazolam, Zolpidem, and Zaleplon

If a patient needs a second dose in the middle of the night to continue consolidated sleep, zaleplon is the drug of choice because of its rapid onset of action and shortest half-life compared to other drugs in this category. It has a short half-life of approximately 1 hour.

Eszopiclone, Oxazepam, Estazolam, Temazepam, and Lorazepam

The drugs with intermediate onset of action and duration of efficacy are eszopiclone, oxazepam, estazolam, temazepam, and lorazepam and are

used for both sleep onset and sleep maintenance insomnia.

Clonazepam, Quazepam, Diazepam, and Flurazepam

Clonazepam, quazepam, diazepam, and flurazepam have a half-life of 23 hours, 39 hours, 43 hours, and 74 hours, respectively. Due to the extremely long half-lives, these are not the ideal drugs for treatment of insomnia as they are effective and can impair daytime functioning and have other side effects. However, they can be appropriately used in patients who have insomnia as well as daytime symptoms of anxiety and who need long-acting anxiolytic therapy.

Clonazepam is considered the standard of therapy for the initial treatment of REM sleep behavior disorder. Its efficacy has been proven, and residual daytime impairment is minimal.

Rebound Insomnia

When discontinued, all the benzodiazepines are known to leave some degree of rebound insomnia. However, the newer benzodiazepine receptor agonists have less incidence of rebound insomnia. Due to the rapid turnover, short-acting benzodiazepines have a greater incidence of rebound insomnia compared to the longer-acting drugs. Rebound insomnia can also be dose dependent; that is, higher doses are likely to cause more chances of rebound insomnia compared to the lower doses of the medication. Of all the available drugs, zopiclone causes the lowest incidence of rebound insomnia. Longer-acting benzodiazepines, with a slow and gradual decline in their blood concentrations, do not cause rebound symptoms when they are withdrawn.

MELATONIN RECEPTOR AGONISTS

Ramelteon

There are two types of melatonin receptors: MT 1 and MT 2. Ramelteon works on both. Currently, it has rapid onset of action and shortness to sleep latency, while increasing total sleep time. Most patients tolerate the drug well due to the low side effect profile. It should be carefully used in patients with liver disease as it is metabolized by the liver.

In addition, it should be carefully used in patients with kidney disease due to its excretion via the kidney. No respiratory depression or drug dependence is known to occur with ramelteon. While using ramelteon, pay careful attention to drug–drug interactions as it can notably increase some side effects of rifampin and decrease the metolazone of alcohol and certain antifungal drugs.

ANTIDEPRESSANTS IN THE TREATMENT OF INSOMNIA

Insomnia and depression can coexist in approximately 60–70% of patients. About one-third of patients with chronic insomnia also developed depression. Insomnia can present 9 months prior to the clinical onset of major depression. Patients with chronic insomnia invariably develop depression. Many available pharmaceutical agents can address both insomnia and depression and should be considered in such a patient population.

Tertiary Tricyclic Antidepressant Drugs (Amitriptyline, Doxepin, Trimipramine)

Tricyclic antidepressant medications have anticholinergic and serotonergic properties. These medications are sedating, and the onset of the sedation effect is immediate. It takes several weeks for the antidepressant effect to occur. Obviously, these drugs also have a significant side effect profile due to their anticholinergic activity.

Trazodone

Trazodone is an interesting medication that is considered the number one drug used by providers in the management of insomnia. This is a non-serotonin reuptake inhibitor (SSRI) antidepressant. Trazodone has anticholinergic, serotonergic, and noradrenergic properties. Its major side effects include cardiac arrhythmias, priapism, and orthostatic hypotension.

Mirtazapine

Mirtazapine has sedating properties along with the antidepressant effect. In some patients, appetite is also improved. It has been used in the treatment of insomnia in patients with coexisting depression and poor appetite.

While using the Tricyclic antidepressants, special attention should be given to the possibility of cardiac arrhythmias, orthostatic hypotension, dry mouth, urinary retention, and blurred vision. These effects can be life-threatening. Many other selective serotonin reuptake inhibitors, including paroxetine, fluoxetine, and sertraline, have been used in patients with coexistent insomnia and depression. Combination therapy has been tried with antidepressants and benzodiazepines. Mild benzodiazepine improves the subjective quality of sleep and does not tend to interfere with the antidepressant effects. Short-acting benzodiazepines such as zaleplon or zolpidem should be considered for this purpose.

TREATMENT FOR EXCESSIVE DAYTIME SLEEPINESS (EDS)

CNS Stimulants

Currently the most common and relatively safer CNS stimulant is modafinil. However, methylphenidate, dextroamphetamine, or other historical stimulants have been used. These agents increase wakefulness and performance, as well as improve the sense of fatigue and tiredness.

Methylphenidate

Methylphenidate increases sleep latency. It is a schedule II medication and needs a prescription. It has multiple side effects, including headaches, insomnia, nervousness, and akathisia, to mention a few.

Dextroamphetamine

Dextroamphetamine is another stimulant that was historically used and is now used occasionally. It has multiple formulations and dosing frequencies. Its major side effects include psychotic behavior, insomnia, and cardiovascular complications.

Modafinil

Modafinil is a rather recently introduced drug that is well tolerated and has mild to moderate side effects. It increases wakefulness during the daytime and reduces daytime sleepiness. It is given in the morning and therefore does not have any effect on nighttime sleep. The most common side effect is headaches, which tend to resolve over time. GI irritation can also occur. Dose modifications are needed in patients with liver disease and advanced age.

Combination Therapy

Combination therapy is desirable, and the patients who have poor response to safer agents like modafinil. However, methylphenidate and dextroamphetamine can be added with increasing doses, and a well-designed titration is scheduled. At this time, the patient may be referred to a sleep specialist or psychiatrist with experience in the use of these drugs. Many psychiatric and psychological conditions like insomnia and psychosis can be precipitated by the long-term use of these medications. If side effects occur, the dose de-escalation should be attempted first.

TREATMENT OF ABNORMAL REM SLEEP INTRUSIONS

REM sleep can include increased fullness, causing symptoms of sleep paralysis or cataplexy. Tricyclic antidepressants are commonly used drugs for managing cataplexy and sleep analysis. Many REM-suppressing medications, including tricyclic antidepressants and selective serotonin reuptake inhibitors, are used effectively for this purpose. Significant withdrawal and rebound symptoms can occur if these medications are suddenly stopped. Despite the potential side effects, tricyclic antidepressants are effective in most patients. If a patient is unable to tolerate the anticholinergic side effects, drugs like fluoxetine should be considered. Again, consider referring the patient to a sleep specialist if initial therapy begins to fail or if side effects begin to occur.

TREATMENT OF CENTRAL SLEEP APNEA CAUSING INSOMNIA

Central sleep apnea manifests as sleep maintenance insomnia. Many therapies have been attempted with variable success rates. While oxygen is used to stabilize ventilation by increasing PCO_2 mildly, it may not work in severe cases. Oxygen therapy in the setting works by Haldane effect affects and blunts the hypoxic ventilatory drive. Another form

of central sleep apnea, Cheyne–Stokes breathing, occurs in patients with congestive heart failure and most commonly after cerebrovascular accidents. It can be treated with Angiotensin-converting enzyme inhibitors, digoxin, diuretics, and beta blockade. Small studies have shown some effective role of methimazole since, adding dead space, acetazolamide, and a variety of positive-airway-pressure-delivered systems.

Methylxanthines

As previously noted, methylxanthines such as theophylline have been reported to improve central sleep apnea and the apnea-hypopnea index within 5 days of treatment in patients with Cheyne–Stokes respiration and congestive heart failure. However, from the primary care perspective, the patient should be referred for further evaluation and be managed by a sleep specialist.

Oxygen

Oxygen by way of the Haldane effect is considered a stabilizer of the breathing pattern in patients with Cheyne–Stokes breathing. It is not known if the oxygen therapy improves daytime symptoms or cardiac performance. While there is much discussion regarding the increase of the dead space or current active therapy, such therapy is not commercially available. Exposure to carbon dioxide for therapeutic purposes is likely to be poorly tolerated and can cause disturbed sleep.

Acetazolamide

The mechanism of action of acetazolamide for use in central sleep apnea is not known. However, it is currently recommended by a few in the high-altitude central sleep apneas and similar medical conditions.

TREATMENT OF PARASOMNIAS

While drug therapy is not the first line of therapy in the treatment of parasomnias, good sleep hygiene, avoiding sleep deprivation of any cause, avoidance of substance use, and the identification and management of underlying sleep disorders causing the parasomnia should be considered first. Mild cases tend to improve with the passage of time especially in children. However, tricyclic antidepressants, benzodiazepines, and paroxetine have been noted to be efficacious in selected patient populations.

PHARMACOLOGIC TREATMENT FOR OBSTRUCTIVE SLEEP APNEA (OSA)

According to the American Academy of Sleep Medicine, the current position of pharmaceutical treatment for obstructive sleep apnea is not optimal. However, pharmaceuticals can be effective as a secondary line of therapy to support positive airway pressure therapy: in this regard, protriptyline, nasal steroids, hormone replacement therapy, and modafinil.

Protriptyline

A number of studies particularly showed variable efficacy in the treatment of obstructive sleep apnea. Selective serotonin rehab uptake inhibitors have also been tested, but no recommendations are available at this time for use of either protriptyline or any selective serotonin reuptake inhibitors (SSRI) for the treatment of obstructive sleep apnea.

Nasal Steroids

Nasal steroid sprays tend to work by reducing the airway obstruction by relieving the congestion of the nasal passage to the airflow. It is also useful for the patient of nasal CPAP who has allergies and other causes of nasal congestion.

Hormone Replacement Therapy

Some studies, including a sleep heart health study, have documented the lower incidence of obstructive sleep apnea. However, currently there is no specific recommendation regarding the use of hormone replacement therapy in the management of obstructive sleep apnea.

Modafinil has been evaluated as an adjunct to CPAP in patients who remain sleepy while being treated with CPAP. It is important to note that this application is limited to those who are actually using and compliant with CPAP.

SLEEPWALKING (SW)

Sleepwalking is a form of parasomnia as previously discussed. The first line of treatment for the same sleepwalking is identification and avoidance of the precipitating causes and securing a safe living space. Safety measures include fire safety, injury due to sharp objects, and locking the door and the windows. In severe cases where the patient is a danger to self or others, some recommendations regarding benzodiazepines and tricyclic antidepressants are available. However, primary care providers should refer these cases to the subspecialist management.

SLEEP TERROR (ST)

Sleep terrors tend to resolve over time, especially in the children. However, if sleep terrors are present in adulthood, it can be a significant problem that needs to be addressed by a sleep specialist, psychologist, or psychiatrist. Clonazepam, trazodone, and paroxetine have been reported to be useful. Again, the primary care provider should consider referring for subspecialty management.

NIGHTMARES

Nightmares are treated only if they are severely refractory. Since nightmares tend to occur during REM sleep, SSRI or tricyclic antidepressant therapy may be useful for REM suppression and therefore the potential decrease in the frequency of nightmares. Unresponsive cases should be referred for subspecialty consultation and management.

REM BEHAVIOR DISORDER (RBD)

REM behavior disorder is a condition when the patients begin to act out their dreams. In most dreams, patients tend to fight an animal predator while trying to save and defend themselves. However, in sleep behavior, they start acting out the fight and hit the bed partner in the process, causing significant injuries. Clonazepam has been considered the first-line medication recommended in most cases. Clonazepam should be considered carefully for patients with kidney problems, respiratory problems, severe liver disease, and glaucoma. Clonazepam should be gradually withdrawn if it has to be discontinued to avoid undesirable symptoms. Difficult cases should be referred for subspecialty evaluation.

RESTLESS LEG SYNDROME (RLS)

Ropinirole or Pramipexole

RLS is a common condition frequently encountered in primary care practice. Dopamine agonists like ropinirole or pramipexole are the first-line treatment. While gabapentin is the secondary therapy, opioids are used in certain patient populations. Benzodiazepines have been used with some success in a few cases.

Dopaminergic Medications

LEVODOPA

Levodopa, while short-acting, can be very effective in resolving RLS symptoms. The real-life disadvantage of levodopa is augmentation, that is, the worsening of symptoms, their increasing intensity and spread to other areas of the body earlier in the day. Augmentation can affect up to 80% of the patients treated with levodopa. The other problem, which can be severe, is rebound; that is, the symptoms tend to occur in the early morning hours and are more intense. Approximately 20–25% patients developed rebound phenomena.

DOPAMINE AGONISTS

Dopamine agonists are currently recommended therapy for the symptomatic control of the RLS. They have much less risk of the augmentation, but the risk of tolerance is high. Pramipexole improves the subjective symptoms of RLS and also improves periodic limb movements while awake. Ropinirole has similar efficacy and is considered the first-line therapy. Rotigotine is another medication used for the same purpose but has significant side effects in susceptible individuals. Apomorphine has been used with fair success in patients with RLS.

ANTICONVULSANTS

Although the mechanism of action of gabapentin in the treatment of RLS is not known, they are the second-line treatment for the patient intolerant to dopamine agonist. It is more effective in patients with renal failure who are dependent on dialysis. Carbamazepine has been effective in some

individuals with RLS. This drug has significant side effects.

OPIOIDS

Finally, opioids are commonly used in the treatment of RLS even when they are considered the third line of treatment. Many patients are intolerant to dopamine agonists and may not be suitable candidates for gabapentin-like medications. Propoxyphene and oxycodone have been used successfully. In addition, methadone does not reduce RLS symptoms. More suitable candidates for methadone therapy would be patients who are poorly responsive to dopamine agonist therapy. Methadone therapy also does not cause augmentation. Long-acting benzodiazepine clonazepam has been successfully used in few patients with RLS.

PRINCIPLES OF PHARMACOLOGIC THERAPY IN PATIENTS WITH SLEEP DISORDERS

While managing patients with sleep disorders with pharmaceutical therapy, it is important to evaluate for the presence of coexistent sleep disorders as disorders present mostly with nonspecific similar symptoms. In difficult cases, the onset of the side effects, or poor response to therapy, primary care providers should have a low threshold to refer the patient for subspecialty consultation.

SUGGESTED READING

1. Pagel JF, Parnes BL. Medications for the treatment of sleep disorders: an overview. *Prim Care Companion J Clin Psychiatry.* 2001;3(3):118–125. http://doi.org/10.4088/pcc.v03n0303
2. Ramar K, Olson EJ. Management of common sleep disorders. *Am Fam Physician.* 2013;88(4):231–238.
3. Holder S, Narula NS. Common sleep disorders in adults: diagnosis and management. *Am Fam Physician.* 2022;105(4):397–405.
4. Dora Zalai MR, Hussain G, Shapiro C. The adult patient with a sleep disorder. In *Psychiatry in Primary Care: A Concise Canadian Pocket Guide*, Canada: CAMH Publications; ISBN: 9781771144193 (print) Product Code: P6516.

25

Simple Positional Devices, Dental Appliances

DEEPAK SHRIVASTAVA, AJITPAL SETHI,
AND RICHA SHRIVASTAVA

POSITIONAL THERAPY IN THE MANAGEMENT OF SNORING AND OTHER OBSTRUCTIVE AIRWAY EVENTS LIKE SLEEP APNEA

Positional therapy treats individuals who sleep in the supine position, causing the obstruction of the airway and leading to a spectrum of symptoms from snoring to obstructive events. A variety of methods are available to avoid assuming the supine position. A night shirt with a back pocket containing a tennis ball, commercially made vests, specially designed pillows, positional alarms, and verbal instructions have been recommended. Multiple studies have demonstrated improvement in intensity, frequency, snoring rate, or duration of the snoring or of obstructive events while using such therapeutic devices. Studies of patients with obstructive sleep apnea have also demonstrated a reduction in the apnea-hypopnea index (AHI) while using positional devices.

A review of the compliance rate with positional therapy indicated that, depending on the type of therapy chosen, the patient may not be able to use the device as recommended. The reasons are discomfort and tightness of the vest around the chest, restless sleep, frequent awakenings, sweating during the night, and inability to resume the preferred and favored sleep position. A few studies have documented lack of effectiveness, back pain, and lack of improvement in the quality of sleep or daytime sleepiness. Not all patients learned to avoid the supine position and either needed continued use or periodic training for reinforcement. Most attended full-night sleep studies called polysomnography (PSG), by which the supine and nonsupine AHI was calculated as a guide in the decision to recommend positional therapy.

DOI: 10.1201/9781003093381-29

Combination therapy for the treatment of obstructive sleep apnea, including continuous positive airway pressure and surgical interventions, according to a few case reports and a small series of reports, suggests that additional positional therapy significantly improved the response to treatment with surgical intervention like uvelopalatopharyngoplasty.

In addition, positional therapy has been evaluated in combination with oral appliance therapy. Patients with position-dependent obstructive sleep apnea receiving positional therapy along with the oral appliance are noted to be more responsive to oral appliance therapy. Reduction in the severity of the obstructive events in the supine position was noted to be the strongest protection of successful combination therapy.

Compliance with the CPAP therapy is relatively poor, and one of the reasons is noted to be high intolerable CPAP pressures. Combination therapy with positional devices has shown a reduction in the required positive pressure to open up the airway and make the CPAP therapy more tolerable. At least one study showed that the compliance in fact improved with the auto-CPAP therapy and that the patient also used a positional device.

As previously noted, commercial products are available that utilize a snowball. Such devices consist of the placement of a number of balls in a pouch attached to the back of the sleepwear. The presence of the ball becomes uncomfortable in the supine position and forces the patient to return to the nonsupine position. Such devices can be handmade at home and could be an inexpensive and easy to use alternative. Sleep position monitors work like a loud alarm if the patient turns on the back. Multiple similar products are available commercially. Products like nasal strips and throat sprays are not the subject of this chapter; however, these are freely available and have variable effects on patients' sleep.

ORAL APPLIANCES IN THE MANAGEMENT OF OBSTRUCTIVE SLEEP APNEA

Overall, appliances are considered first-line therapy for mild to moderate obstructive sleep apnea, just like positive airway pressure. They are also considered in cases of severe sleep apnea when the patient is unable to tolerate and refuses treatment with positive airway pressure devices. Oral appliances are not known to be superior to the different forms of upper airway surgery and seem to be more efficacious. While oral appliances are well tolerated and have a slightly better side effect profile, the efficacy compared to positive airway pressure in the correction of the apnea-hypopnea index is lower. If the disease continues to get worse and takes a severe form or if body weight increases, the efficacy of the oral appliance can decrease. Most of the side effects are minor and can be easily managed.

Types of Oral Appliances

Oral appliances have been used for the treatment of sleep disordered breathing since 1983. Initial oral appliances also used tongue-retaining devices along with mandibular advancement devices. At this time, a number of user-friendly designs have been developed. Multiple different oral appliances are available, and currently 30 appliances have the approval of the Food and Drug Administration (FDA).

Few appliances are approved for snoring only. The oral appliances work by a mechanism where they open the airway by lifting and moving tongue away from the posterior oropharynx and advancing the jaw forward to create more space in the oropharyngeal area. While two basic types of appliances are used, the more common are the mandibular advancement devices, also known as the oral appliances. The tongue-retaining device works by application of suction on the tongue with the pull forward so that it cannot fall back and block the airway. This appliance is not as popular as the manual advancement device/oral appliance.

Mandibular advancement devices are the more common and popular equipment. Recommended devices are custom made, two-piece devices that are attached by a hinge. This device covers the dental arches and forms a rigid monoblock when closed together. Different designs include an icing assembly, hook, strap, wire, or rod to hold the two pieces together. Such a tile design allows the movement of the lower jaw and provides anterior-posterior and occasionally vertical adjustment flexibility.

A few appliances cover only the upper jaw and teeth with a ramp-like portion that extends over the tongue and reaches inferiorly behind the maxillary incisors. When the mouth closes, the mandibular teeth make contact with the ramp and guide the mandible forward as it closes. These appliances are only effective if a patient sleeps with the mouth closed.

Tongue-retaining devices are made out of soft medical-grade silicone and look like a bulb or cavity. The tongue is pushed inside the bulb, which sticks to the tongue. The bulb can also be slightly squeezed in position on the tongue and then released to create a suction force so that it stays attached to the tongue. The suction device can be really helpful in edentulous patients. According to the studies, tongue-retaining devices are not as effective as oral appliances. Patients are also more intolerant to these devices.

Mechanism of Oral Appliances

It is not known how the oral appliances work in opening the airway. It is, however, suspected that the inability to change the current position and therefore increase the oropharyngeal space is the likely mechanical mechanism. It is well-known that sleep disordered breathing occurs at the level of the oropharynx as the most common site of obstruction. Due to the oral appliance's effect on the tongue, as well as the inability to hold the mandible forward, increases the upper airway volume and stabilizes the pharyngeal dilator muscles to decrease the collapsibility of the pharynx. Many people believe that oral appliances increase tone in the genioglossus muscle (the tongue), which also helps to reduce the collapsibility of the pharynx.

Efficacy of Oral Appliances

The current efficacy of the oral appliances is considered to be variable from mild to severe obstructive sleep apnea. It ranges between 76 and 40%, respectively. According to the dental literature, the overall 1 year rate of success as measured by reduction in the apnea-hypopnea index to less than 10 events per hour is found to be 54%. Complete resolution of the apnea-hypopnea index to less than 5 events per hour is noted in approximately 37% of the patients. Oral appliances lower the apnea-hypopnea index and oxygen desaturation events.

Compliance with Oral Appliances

Interestingly, however, compliance with the use of oral appliances is variable from 48 to 84%. These data ranges over 1 year as long-term compliance data are not available. It is suspected that, with the continued use over time, the rate of compliance will go down. According to patient experience, there are multiple reasons for the lower compliance that include discomfort at the jaw, lack of perceived efficacy, or changing over to positive airway pressure therapy. It is also noticed that regular users tend to adjust to the appliances and have less incidence of side effects compared to known users.

Side Effects of Oral Appliances

While compared to positive airway pressure therapy, oral appliances are supposed to be better tolerated; however, minor side effects and complications are experienced by most patients. The complications are transient and improve upon removal of the appliance and tend to become more tolerable over time. Common side effects include temporomandibular joint discomfort, muscle pain, dry mouth, drooling, teeth movement, and soreness. Bite changes can occur and can especially be felt in the morning after removal of the appliance. These appliances can also cause a posterior open bite that is defined as the inability to close on the back teeth. Since oral appliances work by the forward movement of the mandible throughout the night, other teeth are able to contact but back teeth are left open. Various mechanisms are considered implicating the effect of the lateral pterygoid muscle or alterations in the temporomandibular joint capsule. Again, these changes are reversible within a short time after removal of the implants. Still, 10–15% of the patients will suffer with persistent and occasionally pulmonary changes. If complications are severe, then corrections can be made by orthodontic intervention, restorative dentistry, and surgical interventions.

Considering all this, it must be realized that oral appliances provide an alternative to positive airway pressure therapy and prevent the complications related to obstructive sleep apnea. This risk-vs.-benefit ratio should be discussed with the patient so that he can be encouraged to continue using therapy for obstructive sleep apnea.

Treatment Protocol with Oral Appliances

When a patient is referred for an oral appliance after physician referral, a thorough history is obtained by the dental sleep specialist. The sleep-specific history includes signs and symptoms of sleep disordered breathing including snoring, choking episodes, dry mouth and drooling, grinding teeth, and clenching jaw, as well as excessive daytime sleepiness and nocturia. The review of the patient's social life, medications, and lifestyle further increases the pretest probability of establishing a diagnosis. In addition to complete sleep and dental history, a thorough examination of the face, oropharynx, and maxillofacial region is performed. Special attention is given to the temporomandibular joint and the dentition. The examination also includes assessment of the masticatory muscles, range of motion of muscle, bruxism-related damage, and assessment of the perioral soft tissues. Intraoral films further provide information along with the cephalogram. Review of the available sleep studies is further helpful in making a decision regarding the eligibility of the patient for the oral appliance therapy.

Relative Contraindications for Oral Appliance Therapy

- Only few teeth present
- Short crowns over teeth
- Poor oral health and periodontal disease
- TMJ diseases
- A prohibitive gag reflex
- Children with continued craniofacial growth

Predictors of Successful Outcomes

- Women
- Mild sleep disordered breathing
- Supine-position-dependent obstructive sleep apnea
- Ability to move mandible forward

Predictors of Suboptimal Outcomes

- Severe cases of obstructive sleep apnea
- Morbid obesity
- Nasal congestion and increased resistance to nasal airflow

Selection of Oral Appliance

Multiple factors need to be considered before selecting an oral appliance for a particular patient. Some of the patient-related factors include complaints of bruxism, the actual number and condition of the teeth, the inability to move the jaw and temporal mandibular joint, and patient willingness to proceed.

Appliance-related factors include the availability of the most recommended two-piece appliance attached with a hinge, ease of use, and adjustability of the appliance.

The education, American Academy of Dental Sleep Medicine (AADSM) certification, and experience of the dentist play an important role in the success of the oral appliance therapy.

Initial Assessment and Preparation

The dentist generally would assess a patient's protrusive range and subsequently obtain a bite recording based on the comfortable protruded position of the jaw. This position generally lies between 50 and 75% of the patient's movement range. Once the impressions are obtained, the bite records are forwarded to the fabrication lab.

Initial Fitting of the Oral Appliance

Once fabricated and individualized, oral appliances are received, and the initial fitting is done in the dental office. The patient is monitored over a number of weeks with minor adjustments made in order to find the most beneficial and comfortable position for the patient. At this stage, a follow-up sleep study is not done; the patient's subjective reports of improvement in symptoms guides the treatment decision. Many dentists use a type III study during this process.

Final Fitting and Follow-up

Once the patient reports resolution of their symptoms and the lack of any side effects at that time in-lab, polysomnography can be performed with titration of the oral appliance done by a specialized sleep lab technician who follows the titration protocol provided by the dental sleep specialist. The patient is regularly followed up by the dental sleep specialist in order to recognize any complications and to troubleshoot. According to the current recommendation, a patient is seen by the dental sleep specialist on a 6-month basis and a medical sleep specialist on yearly basis.

According to the American Academy of Dental Sleep Medicine and American Academy of Sleep Medicine (AASM) guidelines, oral appliances are considered first-line therapy for mild to moderate sleep apnea and should be used in cases of severe sleep apnea if the patient is either intolerant or refuses positive airway pressure therapy. Most of the side effects that occur are transient and resolve over time.

SUGGESTED READING

1. Dieltjens M, Vanderveken O. Oral appliances in obstructive sleep apnea. *Healthcare (Basel)*. 2019;7(4):141. http://doi.org/10.3390/healthcare7040141.

2. Marklund M, Braem MJA, Verbraecken J. Update on oral appliance therapy. *Eur Respir Rev*. 2019;28:19008.

3. Ramar K, Dort LC, Katz SG, et al. Clinical practice guideline for the treatment of obstructive sleep apnea and snoring with oral appliance therapy: an update for 2015. *J Clin Sleep Med*. 2015;11:773–827.

4. Sharples LD, Clutterbuck-James AL, Glover MJ, et al. Meta-analysis of randomized controlled trials of oral mandibular advancement devices and continuous positive airway pressure for obstructive sleep apnea-hypopnoea. *Sleep Med Rev*. 2016;27:108–124.

26

Titration Protocols, Continuous Positive Airway Pressure (CPAP), and Other PAP Devices

DEEPAK SHRIVASTAVA, AND AJITPAL SETHI

DETERMINING THE OPTIMAL CPAP SETTING

In order to determine the most appropriate CPAP pressure that would be tolerated by the patient and that will resolve all episodes of obstructive events, including apneas, hypopneas, respiratory-effort-related arousals, and snoring, and that will stabilize oxygen desaturation, the patient generally goes through a CPAP titration. Overnight CPAP titration has been historically recommended; however, it is unpopular due to the minimum of 2 nights to be spent in the sleep lab. Instead, patients may prefer a split-night study on the same night of the diagnostic study to allow for titration and the complete process with the CPAP prescription. Some data suggest the use of AutoPAP therapy to determine the appropriate CPAP pressure, which is variable based on the body position and resistance to flow and pressure, to be recommended. However, there are no specific guidelines at this time to the support use of AutoPAP as a surrogate for CPAP titration. Conceptually, however, this appears to be a good option to combine a type III study with the AutoPAP in order to establish a diagnosis and treatment of obstructive sleep apnea. Given the high prevalence of sleep disordered breathing, this may be a future intervention available for a selected subset of patients.

Split-night Sleep Study

A split-night sleep study is supported by many third-party payers and is preferred by patients as they have to spend only one night in the sleep lab away

DOI: 10.1201/9781003093381-30

from home. The split-night sleep study documents the obstructive events including apneas and hypopneas according to the specimen guidelines provided by the American Academy of Sleep Medicine. These include an AHI of 20–40 events per hour during the initial 2 hours of the sleep study that qualifies the patient to proceed with the CPAP titration part of the study. A duration of 3 hours must be available in order to titrate the CPAP therapy. If the CPAP titration cannot be completed, a second night of full titration study should be considered.

AASM Criteria for Split-night Sleep Study

- AHI of $\geq$ 40 events/hour during the first 2 hours of the sleep study
- At least 3 hours available to complete a CPAP titration

A variety of improvements have been made over the continuous positive airway pressure in order to increase patient comfort and efficacy of positive airway pressure therapy. This therapy includes levels of pressure on his BiPAP, automatic adjustment machines known as AutoPap and features like extra pressure relief.

BILEVEL POSITIVE PRESSURE THERAPY (BIPAP)

BiPAP therapy provides two different levels of pressure. During inspiration, a high level of pressure applied to open the airway is known as inspiratory positive airway pressure (IPAP); during exhalation, the patient is allowed to breathe out again at a lower pressure, known as expiratory positive airway pressure (EPAP). The difference between the two pressures is the pressure support. This pressure keeps the airway open throughout the respiratory cycle. Despite this improvement, BiPAP therapy has not been proven to be more acceptable to the patient population, and compliance has remained the same. Multiple BiPAP systems have been introduced with unique proprietary features in order to manipulate the application of pressure or the flow to increase patient comfort.

EXPIRATORY PRESSURE RELIEF SYSTEMS (EPR)

Expiratory pressure relief (EPR) was developed in order to improve a patient's ability to exhale against the positive pressure. In EPR mode, the pressure is briefly reduced during the expiration cycle of the breath to give a sense of comfort to the patient before the next respiratory breath is given. The pressure relief is calculated by many parameters including patient effort and the airflow and is variable from one breath to the other. At least 2–3 different levels of pressure relief options are available according to the patient's comfort. These algorithms are proprietary and are variable among different brands of the equipment.

> In an initial nonrandomized study that followed 89 CPAP-naive OSAS patients over a 3 month period, patients using the C-Flex technology demonstrated improved compliance compared with those using fixed-pressure CPAP therapy. In fact, after 3 months of treatment, compliance with C-Flex therapy was greater by an average of 1.7 hours per night. Subjective sleepiness and objective outcomes were similar between the groups. While these initial results were intriguing, the study was limited by its nonrandomized design.
>
> A randomized control trial of C-Flex technology evaluated 52 CPAP-naive patients with newly diagnosed OSAS and allocated them to either fixed CPAP or C-Flex therapy. All patients in the C-Flex group were treated with a C-Flex setting of 3. After 7 weeks of treatment, both CPAP and C-Flex groups demonstrated equal objective compliance (5.2 and 5.3 hours, respectively). Both treatments also demonstrated equal improvements in subjective daytime sleepiness and reductions in the AHI. Finally, C-Flex therapy offered no significant benefits in that subgroup of patients who required pressures of ≥ 9 cm H_2O.

Like other improvements and features that are designed to increase patient comfort, the C-Flex technology did not increase the patient compliance for usage or any other outcomes in another randomized trial.

AUTOMATIC PAP (APAP)

AutoPAP therapy is based on the principles of detecting the flow of the air and the resistance to the flow in real-time and adjusting the pressure accordingly to maintain a certain flow and keep the airway open. Most APAP machines utilize the flow-based algorithm. The arthrogram identifies changes in the inspiratory flow pattern and is directly measured by the patient from snoring, and inspiratory flow limitation. When the sensor recognizes the impedance to flow, the AutoPAP device is programmed to increase the levels of pressure until a preset flow is reached and breathing is normalized. The AutoPAP range on such a device is set at 4–20 cm of water pressure. In many situations where CPAP titration is not possible, AutoPAP technology is really helpful and provides the needed service to the patient.

The AASM committee has recommended that APAP devices not be used in the following groups of patients, and they should not be titrated with an APAP device that relies on vibration or sound in the device's algorithm:

- Congestive heart failure
- Lung diseases such as COPD
- Patients expected to have nocturnal arterial oxyhemoglobin desaturation owing to conditions other than OSAS (e.g., obesity hypoventilation syndrome).
- Patients who do not snore (either naturally or because they have undergone palatal surgery)

APAP devices are not used for split-night titrations given the lack of data to support such a practice.

GOALS FOR POSITIVE AIRWAY PRESSURE TITRATION

Positive airway pressure titration is designed to reduce obstructive events, including apneas, hypopneas, respiratory-effort-related arousals, snoring, and resolved oxygen desaturation. Titration protocol is provided by the American Academy of Sleep Medicine to be used in the sleep labs.

CPAP TITRATION PROTOCOLS (AASM PROTOCOL SUMMARIZED)

1. Start a pressure 5 cm H_2O (may start higher pressure for obesity or for re-titration studies).

2. Increase inspiratory pressure to resolve all apneas, hypopneas, RERAs, and snoring.
3. Increase pressure at least by 1 cm H_2O, no sooner than every 5 minutes (for at least 2 obstructive apneas, or at least 3 hypopneas, or at least 5 RERAs, or at least 3 minutes of loud or unambiguous snoring).
4. Exploration pressure may increase 2–5 cm to overcome upper airway resistance to normalize the shape of the inspiratory flow limitation,
5. Down titration is not necessary.
6. If patients are still hypoxic after respiratory events are resolved, do not increase pressure. Maximum CPAP pressure—15 cm H_2O.

All patients tried with nasal CPAP must have a pre-polysomnogram clinical diagnosis of obstructive sleep apnea.

Nasal CPAP will not be performed on patients who have a recent history of any of the following conditions unless approved by the clinical polysomnographer or medical director:

- Bullous lung disease
- Pneumothorax
- Low blood pressure (i.e., systolic BP < 90 mm Hg and/or clinical signs and symptoms of inadequate perfusion)

A therapeutic trial of nasal CPAP will be instituted the same night as the initial polysomnogram if the following criteria are met (any deviation from this protocol must be approved by the medical director or clinical polysomnographer):

- The patient has a pre-polysomnogram clinical diagnosis of obstructive sleep apnea.
- The clinical polysomnographer or medical director has reviewed the clinical history and approved the combined diagnostic/CPAP trials.
- During the polysomnogram recording, the technologist observes either:
  - Frequent episodes of obstructive apneas/hypopneas (>30/hour), or
  - Oxygen saturation by oximetry repeatedly falls to or below 85%.

- It is preferred to postpone the CPAP trial until the first REM period has occurred, but this is not necessary if there is sufficient evidence of obstructive sleep apnea and there is limited time remaining to conduct a CPAP trial.
- The patient has been informed of the nasal CPAP procedure.

PROCEDURAL PROTOCOL

- The procedure for performing a polysomnogram with nasal continuous positive airway pressure (CPAP) is consistent with the nocturnal polysomnogram procedure.
- Prior to the procedure, the patient will be given an explanation of the procedure by the technologist.
- The CPAP pressure is to be monitored continuously throughout the study using a clinical remote.
- Begin the pressure titration at 3–5 cm H_2O. Observe for apneas, hypopneas, oxygen desaturations, snoring, and respiratory arousals. Upon observation of any one of these particulars, increase the pressure in an increment of 1–2 cm H_2O. (Subsequent occurrences of any of these particulars will warrant additional pressure increases.)

Allow the patient to adjust to any increase in pressure for at least 10 minutes. Monitor the continuance of apneas, hypopneas, oxygen desaturations, snoring, and/or respiratory arousals. If the patient continues to present with any of these findings, the pressure may be increased after 10 minutes in increments of 1–2 cm H_2O.

The final CPAP pressure is obtained upon resolution of respiratory obstructions, oxygen desaturations, snoring, and respiratory arousals in all body positions and stages of sleep.

Heated humidification can be added as needed to patients using high CPAP pressures, patients complaining of nasal congestion, and/or dryness or nasal irritation.

The patient may be given a nasal mask if it is available. Patients will be provided with information on the different CPAP equipment that is available and a list of approved home health care companies (unless directed otherwise by a referring physician). Patients will be provided with discharge instructions that are explained to the patient by the technologists when they leave the sleep center.

BILEVEL PAP TITRATION (AASM PROTOCOL SUMMARIZED)

According to the American Academy of Sleep Medicine, BiPAP should be used in patients who are intolerant to the high pressure of CPAP. The other criterion is that, if a patient continues to have apneas, hypopneas, and respiratory-effort-related arousals at a CPAP pressure of 15 cm of water during the titration study, the titration should be switched to BiPAP therapy. The difference of 4 cm of water pressure was maintained between the inspiratory and expiratory pressures. The maximum difference can be no more than 10 cm of water pressure.

Expiratory Pressure Relief

Expiratory pressure relief of 20% can be used in order to offset the subjective feeling of exhaling against high pressure. It is likely to improve patient comfort but has not been proven to improve patient compliance.

TITRATION PROTOCOL FOR AUTO-CPAP (CPAP <10 CMH2O)

- Set AutoMin at 4 cmH_2O or patient comfort
- Set AutoMax to 20 cmH_2O
- Set A-Flex to patient comfort

TITRATION PROTOCOL FOR AUTO-CPAP (CPAP >10 CMH2O)

- Set AutoMin at 6–8 cm H_2O or patient comfort.
- Set AutoMax to 20 cm H_2O.
- Set A-Flex to patient comfort.

Indication for APAP

- Uncomplicated moderate to severe OSAS
- REM-related OSAS
- Position dependence
- High pressures (>10)
- CPAP-intolerant patients

- Congestive heart failure
- COPD and chronic lung disease
- Obesity hypoventilation syndrome
- Other hypoventilation syndromes
- Lack of snoring

CPAP TITRATION ALGORITHM FOR PATIENTS ≥12 YEARS DURING FULL- OR SPLIT-NIGHT TITRATION STUDIES

The following is the American Academy of Sleep Medicine summary of the CPAP titration algorithm for patients ≥12 years during full or split-night titration studies. It has been modified from the AASM practice parameters:

- Upward titration at ≥1 cm increments over ≥ 5-minute periods is continued according to the breathing events observed until ≥30 minutes without breathing events is achieved.
- A higher starting CPAP may be selected for patients with an elevated BMI and for re-titration studies.
- The patient should also be tried on BIPAP if the patient is uncomfortable or intolerant of high CPAP.

BPAP TITRATION ALGORITHM FOR PATIENTS ≥12 YEARS DURING FULL- OR SPLIT-NIGHT TITRATION STUDIES

The following is the American Academy of Sleep Medicine summary of the BPAP titration algorithm for patients ≥12 years during full or split-night titration studies:

- Upward titration of IPAP and EPAP ≥1 cm H_2O for apneas and IPAP ≥1 cm for other events over ≥5 minute periods is continued until ≥30 minutes without breathing events is achieved.

- A decrease in IPAP or setting BPAP in spontaneous timed mode with the backup rate may be helpful if treatment-emergent central apneas are observed.
- A higher starting IPAP and EPAP may be selected for patients with an elevated BMI and for re-titration studies.
- When transitioning from CPAP to BIPAP, the minimum starting EPAP should be set at 4 cm H_2O or the CPAP level at which obstructive apneas were eliminated. An optimal minimum IPAP-EPAP differential is 4 cm H_2O, and an optimal maximum IPAP-EPAP differential is 10 cm H_2O.

SUGGESTED READING

1. Patil SP, Ayappa IA, Caples SM, et al. Treatment of adult obstructive sleep apnea with positive airway pressure: an American Academy of Sleep Medicine Clinical practice guideline. *J Clin Sleep Med.* 2019;15:335.
2. Kushida CA, Chediak A, Berry RB, Brown LK, Gozal D, Iber C, Parthasarathy S, Quan SF, Rowley JA. Positive airway pressure titration task force of the American Academy of Sleep Medicine: clinical guidelines for the manual titration of positive airway pressure in patients with obstructive sleep apnea. *J Clin Sleep Med.* 2008;4(2):157–171.
3. Al Zuheibi T, Al Abri M. Effects of three modes of respironics auto CPAP machines in patients with OSAHS. *Sleep Med.* 2013;14(S1):e316–e317.
4. https://cpapsupplies.com/blog/flex-c-flex-epr-whats-difference
5. Marcus CL, Beck SE, Traylor J, Cornaglia MA, Meltzer LJ, DiFeo N, Karamessinis LR, Samuel J, Falvo J, DiMaria M, Gallagher PR, Beris H, Menello MK. Randomized, double-blind clinical trial of two different modes of positive airway pressure therapy on adherence and efficacy in children. *J Clin Sleep Med.* 2012;8(1):37–42.

PART 5

Self-Assessment

27

Chapter-Based Assessment

KARUNA DATTA, AND DEEPAK SHRIVASTAVA

INTRODUCTION

This chapter helps the reader assess the knowledge acquired by answering questions framed from the concepts brought out in this book. After going through the chapters in the book, taking these questions may be an excellent way for a quick recapitulation too. There are a total of 55 questions, and the answers are listed in the "Solutions" section at the end of this chapter. After each correct answer is a reference to the chapter number(s) where the concept was covered in detail.

This assessment is specifically planned as a learning tool to help the reader assimilate the basic concepts of sleep medicine. The questions are framed at a very basic level and are not restricted to just recall type but have a mix of case-based scenarios and other types that enable the reader to reach the comprehension level in the cognitive domain of learning. Though basic concepts are targeted here, but unless these concepts are clear, it is very difficult to comprehend questions based on the higher cognitive domains of analysis and evaluation for sleep medicine practice.

It is also imperative to state here that the multiple-choice questions are built around concepts and not made specifically for any competition, grading exams, etc. The answer given for a particular question need not be the only correct one but is rather the best choice for the given set of distractors.

Hence it should not be confusing if the same choice in another question with different distractors may not be the only answer or the best one.

DIRECTIONS

The following questions are best-response, multiple-choice questions. Each question is followed by four distractors. Mark the best response as the answer. Questions that prompt multiple responses may be responded to accordingly. The answer key for all the questions is given at the end of the section.

Case: A 15-year-old reports with a history of going to bed at 11 p.m. He does his pending schoolwork till 2 a.m. and then decides to sleep. He sleeps immediately after lying in bed and then gets up at around 11a.m. Because there is a lot of activity in the morning hours at home, he is unable to sleep well in the morning hours. This has been his habit for 2 years, ever since the pandemic struck. Since his school has gone online, most days he would get up at 8.30 a.m., log in the attendance, and then try to attend school but would doze off intermittently. He preferred to sleep uninterrupted till 11 a.m. His school was online all this while, but now he needs to go offline. He recently tried going to bed early for 2–3 days but complains that he could not sleep and just kept on tossing and turning in bed till 2 a.m. and only after that he could sleep. There is no

DOI: 10.1201/9781003093381-32

other evidence of any other comorbidity or any other complaints.

1. What is he most likely suffering from?
   a) Acute sleep deprivation
   b) Delayed sleep-wake phase syndrome
   c) Chronic insomnia
   d) Irregular sleep-wake rhythm disorder
2. How would you assess this patient?
   a) An overnight polysomnography with 2 week sleep diary
   b) 2 week sleep diary, thought diary, dreams diary, and an overnight polysomnography
   c) 2 week sleep diary and an overnight actigraphy
   d) 2 week sleep diary initially
3. What should be the first line of treatment for this patient?
   a) Asking him to follow from the first day to lie in bed and try sleeping at 10 a.m. and instructing parents to ensure switching on his bedroom lights in the morning the next day onward and drawing back the curtains at around 4–5 a.m..
   b) Postawakening light therapy, behavioral intervention following sleep hygiene principles, and try switching the bedtime from 2 a.m. to 12 midnight slowly in a couple of days and then reassessing after 2 weeks.
   c) Initially only sharing with him the pamphlet about sleep hygiene principles to motivate him to follow them since the first step of treatment is self-motivation alone and asking him to report after 1 month.
   d) Asking him to go to bed at 10 p.m. after taking zolpidem such that he can sleep on time from that very night, causing the distress to be reduced immediately.

Case: A 75-year-old patient reports with the inability to stay awake during evening time. His history revealed that he had 3 sons and that they were residing with him with their families. The entire family would have dinner together at 8.30 p.m. He had the complaint that he felt very guilty at times as he would eat at 7 p.m. and go off to sleep before family dinner time. On further exploring, it was clear that he was having this problem for the past 1–2 years and was almost every day now, which was creating a kind of concern for him since he felt left out from family time. He also would

wake up around 3 a.m. and start his morning routine. This was also a problem for him since his sons feared that he is alone while exercising and walking around the house and would recommend that he sleep or stay in his room safely.

4. What is he most likely to be suffering from?
   a) Advanced sleep-wake phase syndrome
   b) Delayed sleep-wake phase syndrome
   c) Chronic insomnia
   d) Irregular sleep-wake rhythm disorder
5. How would you like to assess this patient?
   a) An overnight polysomnography with 2 week sleep diary
   b) 2 week sleep diary, thought diary, dreams diary, and an overnight polysomnography
   c) 2 week sleep diary and an overnight actigraphy
   d) 2 week sleep diary initially
6. What should be the first line of treatment for this patient?
   a) Asking him from the first day to try to sleep and lie in bed until 5a.m. and instructing family members to ensure that he does so.
   b) Timed light therapy in the evening and a short nap in the afternoon.
   c) Initially only sharing with him the pamphlet about sleep hygiene principles to motivate him to follow them since the first step of treatment is self-motivation alone and asking him to report after 1 month.
   d) Asking him to lie in bed after taking zolpidem at 3a.m. so that he can sleep until at least 5a.m. from that very night, causing the distress to reduce immediately.
7. A patient complains of daytime sleepiness and not feeling refreshed after waking up. On history taking, he says that for the past 7 months, he has been sleeping without any difficulty, every night regularly at around 12.30 a.m., and waking up at 6:00 a.m. What is he most likely suffering from?
   a) Delayed sleep-wake phase syndrome
   b) Paradoxical insomnia
   c) Chronic insomnia
   d) Sleep deprivation
8. A 38-year-old patient reports to the outpatient department with a history of sleep complaints for past 2 years. He goes to bed to sleep regularly at 10 p.m. and wakes up at 6 a.m., but he takes 30–45 minutes to sleep initially after

going to bed to sleep. This happens almost every day of the week. He also complains of associated daytime dysfunction due to this problem of reduced concentration and attention during work at office. What is his primary problem likely to be?

a) Delayed sleep-wake phase syndrome
b) Paradoxical insomnia
c) Chronic insomnia
d) Insufficient sleep syndrome

9. Which of the following is NOT a NREM or REM parasomnia?

a) Periodic limb movement disorder
b) Sleep terrors
c) Sleep talking
d) Confusional arousals

10. *Pavor nocturnus* refer to which of the following sleep disorders?

a) Periodic limb movement disorder
b) Sleep terrors
c) Sleep talking
d) Confusional arousals

11. An important differentiating feature between sleep deprivation and insomnia is:

a) wake-up time
b) providing adequate opportunity to sleep
c) associated daytime dysfunction
d) duration of sleep complaints

12. CBT_{min}, is the time at which the core body temperature is the minimum. It generally occurs:

a) 3–4 hours before habitual bedtime
b) 3–4 hours after habitual bedtime
c) 3–4 hours before habitual wake-up time
d) 3–4 hours after habitual wake-up time

13. A patient habitually sleeps at 11 p.m. and wakes up at 7 a.m. Keeping the phase response curve of circadian rhythm to light, the best response to advance the sleep phase would occur when light exposure occurs at:

a) 6–8 p.m.
b) 10 p.m.–12 midnight
c) 6–8 a.m.
d) 10 a.m.–12 noon

14. The likelihood of developing jet lag syndrome as compared to eastward travel vs. westward travel, is more if the:

a) eastward travel is more than 2 time zones
b) eastward travel is less than 2 time zones
c) westward travel is more than 2 time zones
d) westward travel is less than 2 time zones

15. Which of the following is NOT a recommended drug of choice for sleep onset insomnia?

a) Triazolam
b) Temazepam
c) Eszopiclone
d) Melatonin

16. Which of the following is NOT a recommended drug of choice for sleep maintenance insomnia?

a) Suvorexant
b) Temazepam
c) Eszopiclone
d) Melatonin

17. Which of the following is a recommended drug of choice for sleep onset insomnia?

a) Zolpidem
b) Diphenhydramine
c) Melatonin
d) Valerian

18. Which of the following is a recommended drug of choice for sleep maintenance insomnia?

a) Zolpidem
b) Diphenhydramine
c) Melatonin
d) Valerian

19. Home sleep apnea testing is recommended only if the pretest STOP-BANG Questionnaire score is

a) >2
b) >3
c) >5
d) >8

20. Home sleep apnea testing is most likely to be recommended for a case of OSA

a) suggestive of increased risk of moderate to severe OSA
b) with hypoventilation
c) with prior sleep apnea surgery
d) with COPD

21. On a polysomnography trace, the progressive increased effort to breathe in the setting of declining flow eventually causing cortical arousal and awakening of the patient with no oxygen desaturation is called

a) hypopnea
b) apnea
c) RERA
d) mixed apnea

22. On a polysomnography trace, a cessation of airflow from the nose and mouth and absence

of diaphragmatic and abdominal efforts lasting 10 seconds or longer, even without desaturation, is called
a) central apnea
b) obstructive apnea
c) mixed apnea
d) RERA

23. Which of the following is a predictor of a successful outcome of oral appliance therapy?
a) Pronounced gag reflex
b) Supine-dependent apnea in a male
c) Few teeth with short clinical crowns
d) Moderate OSA

24. Which of the following is a part of the polysomnography diagnostic criteria for periodic limb movement disorder in an adult?
a) Periodic limb movements are scored if they are part of a series of 4 or more consecutive movements lasting 5–10 seconds, with an intermovement interval of 90–150 seconds and a PLMS index of >5 movements per hour of sleep.
b) Periodic limb movements are scored if they are part of a series of 4 or more consecutive movements lasting 0.5–5 seconds, with an intermovement interval of 4–90 seconds and a PLMS index of >15 movements per hour of sleep.
c) Periodic limb movements are scored if they are part of a series of 4 or more consecutive movements lasting 0.5–5 seconds, with an intermovement interval of 60–150 seconds and a PLMS index of >15 movements per hour of sleep.
d) Periodic limb movements are scored if they are part of a series of 4 or more consecutive movements lasting 5–35 seconds, with an intermovement interval of 90–150 seconds and a PLMS index of >15 movements per hour of sleep.

25. Patients on polysomnography show a state of partial awakening, slow mentation, disorientation, perceptual impairment, and errors of logic. The memory for the event is often absent. The event may last several minutes and typically happens in the first one-third of night. What is the likely diagnosis?
a) REM parasomnia
b) Sleep paralysis following sleep deprivation
c) Confusional arousal
d) REM behavior disorder

26. The multiple sleep latency test (MSLT) is an objective sleep latency test for sleepiness. It gives a mean sleep latency, which is a measure of the physiologic propensity for sleep in the absence of alerting factors. Which of the following is true about this test?
a) Five nap opportunities are given in the afternoon immediately after the overnight sleep night study night.
b) Each nap period may last for 15 minutes, if sleep is demonstrated on the EEG.
c) MSLT always correlates well with the Epworth Sleepiness Scale.
d) MSLT should be done in the morning hours and only before the polysomnography night.

27. Which of the following is least likely to report with excessive daytime sleepiness?
a) Insufficient sleep syndrome
b) Severe OSA
c) Rotational shift worker
d) Paradoxical insomnia

28. The respiratory drive to the carbon dioxide concentration is most sensitive during the:
a) Wake state
b) NREM state
c) REM state
d) Both the wake and REM states

29. CPAP or BIPAP compliance is better when using EPR. EPR stands for:
a) expiratory pressure at rest
b) expiratory pressure release
c) end pressure relaxation
d) end pneumatic dilation

30. A provision for a backup rate to provide a minimum number of breaths if a patient is unable to take spontaneous breaths is available with which of the following?
a) Spontaneous/timed BiPAP
b) Spontaneous option in BiPAP
c) CPAP
d) AutoPAP

31. When a patient is sensitive to pressure, the ramp feature allows CPAP to start:
a) at a lower pressure and move gradually to the prescribed pressure, once the subject is asleep over a period of time.
b) immediately helps with the prescribed pressure and then, once the patient is comfortable, gets the pressure lower.

c) at a continuous prescribed pressure without reducing or increasing the pressure.

d) at a higher pressure than prescribed until the patient is comfortably asleep, after which it is reduced to keep the patient comfortable while asleep.

32. BiPAP provides assistance during the:
a) inspiratory phase and prevents airway closure during the expiratory phase
b) expiratory phase and prevents airway closure during inspiratory phase
c) inspiratory phase and prevents airway closure also during this phase
d) expiratory phase and prevents airway closure also during this phase

33. Which of the following is NOT recommended to improve snoring for patients who snore?
a) cessation of smoking, reduced alcohol consumption, and improving sleep hygiene
b) myofunctional therapy
c) positional therapy
d) sedatives

34. A 5-year-old child is brought to the family doctor with complaints of occasionally sleepwalking at night. The mother said that this is a recent development and noticed that the child was sleepwalking. This happened when the mother was retiring to bed after completing all the household chores, approximately 1–1.5 hours after the child had gone off to sleep. He was snoring too and on examination showed nasal congestion. The mother had never seen this kind of an episode earlier though she always goes to sleep much later than the child and is generally available to notice in case the child showed any abnormal activity at that time. As a primary care physician, what should be your initial response?
a) Immediately refer for an overnight polysomnography and ask the patient to come once the report is available.
b) Advise the mother to make the bedroom safe, remove all sharp objects, place the child's bed on the floor, and prescribe medications for nasal allergy and advice for an otorhinolaryngolist opinion and to report back after that.
c) Prescribe nasal congestants and reassure the mother that she should not worry at all.

d) Reassure the mother and refer the child to the neurologist immediately.

35. Which of the following is a sleep quality assessment questionnaire?
a) PSQI
b) DBAS
c) STOP-BANG
d) DASS

36. Which of the following is a sleep apnea assessment questionnaire?
a) PSQI
b) DBAS
c) STOP-BANG
d) DASS

37. Which of the following questionnaires assesses various sleep and insomnia-related cognitions?
a) PSQI
b) DBAS
c) STOP-BANG
d) DASS

38. Results have proven that usage of nasal CPAP in most cases improves:
a) atrial fibrillation
b) hypertension
c) sleep quality
d) neurological deterioration in stroke

39. Which of the following is a contraindication for APAP?
a) Uncomplicated moderate to severe OSAS
b) REM-related OSAS
c) CPAP-intolerant patients
d) Lack of snoring

40. Which of the following regulates PER stability by inhibiting post-translational nuclear translocation of PER protein and tags it for degradation by phosphorylating them?
a) CK1ε
b) CRY
c) BMAL
d) CLOCK

41. Which of the following can couple the peripheral clock from the master clock?
a) Social cues
b) Feeding time
c) Light exposure
d) Activity state

42. Sympathetic stimulation of the heart causes (tick one or more choices):
a) increased bathmotropic effect
b) increased dromotropic effect

c) increased lusitropic effect

d) increased ionotropic effect

43. Non-demand myocardial infarction seen in patients with significant endothelial dysfunction would be seen in:
    a) REM sleep
    b) NREM sleep
    c) Wake state during mild exercise
    d) Wake state during moderate to severe exercise

44. The predilection for cardiac events during NREM sleep is due to all of the following conditions EXCEPT:
    a) increased prothrombotic milieu during sleep
    b) endothelial dysfunction
    c) reduced sympathetic activity
    d) increased velocity of blood flow

45. A case with a long history of abnormal movements at night and abnormal behavior during sleep witnessed by a bed partner reports as an outpatient. Which of the following instructions will you give to the sleep technician conducting the overnight polysomnography? (Tick one or more responses.)
    a) The technician should be in attendance in the sleep lab especially in the first half of the night.
    b) Place an extended EEG montage and side rails to the sleep lab bed for safety.
    c) Conduct a split-night polysomnography on the first night itself even in the absence of an earlier polysomnography.
    d) Completely video-record the study.

46. For the data analysis, software in the actigraph uses which of the following for actigraphy report? (Tick one or more responses.)
    a) Time above threshold (TAT), which uses the amount of time per epoch that the activity is above a defined threshold.
    b) Zero crossing mode (ZCM), which counts the number of times per epoch that the signal crosses zero.
    c) Light intensity data, which is the area under the curve for light above a threshold value.
    d) The directions in which the non-dominant arm is moved on which the actigraph is placed.

47. Which of the following is NOT an indication for an actigraphy alone?
    a) Diagnosis of PLMD
    b) Diagnosis of CRSWD

c) OSA (when integrated with HSAT)

d) Estimate TST in sleep deprivation

48. If the sleep efficiency is lower than 85%, and TST is 5.5 hours, which of the following components of CBTI is not recommended?
    a) Relaxation
    b) Cognitive restructuring
    c) Stimulus control
    d) Sleep restriction

49. Light therapy is NOT recommended for patients with:
    a) advanced sleep-wake phase disorder in the elderly
    b) irregular sleep-wake disorder in the elderly combined with melatonin
    c) jet lag disorder
    d) shift work disorder

50. In a counselling session, the counsellor aims to:
    a) change the behavior of the counselee
    b) modify the thinking patterns of the counselee
    c) modify the beliefs of the counselee that hamper health
    d) help the individual to identify the problem and formulate his own strategy to cope with issues

51. Which of the following has/have the most sedating effects?
    a) Desipramine
    b) Nortriptylline
    c) Doxepin
    d) Imipramine

52. Fluoxetine, a SSRI is most likely to cause:
    a) reduced slow wave sleep
    b) increased REM latency
    c) increased REM sleep
    d) reduced N1 sleep

53. A patient of OSA, compliant with CPAP as obtained subjectively, objectively, and from family verification, still complains of daytime sleepiness. The recommended line of treatment would be to add:
    a) both methylphenidate and dextroamphetamine initially
    b) modafinil and, if patient doesn't respond, then methylphenidate
    c) dextroamphetamine and, if patient doesn't respond, then add modafinil
    d) modafinil and, if patient doesn't respond, then add dextroamphetamine

54. Which of the following drug worsens restless leg syndrome?
    a) fluoxetine
    b) ropinirole
    c) pramipexole
    d) levodopa
55. Which of the following drugs is most likely to cause rebound insomnia on withdrawal?
    a) fluoxetine
    b) doxepin
    c) suvorexant
    d) alprazolam

SOLUTIONS

1. b), refer to Chapters 13 and 14
2. d), refer to Chapter 13
3. b), refer to Chapter 13
4. a), refer to Chapters 13 and 14
5. d), refer to Chapter 13
6. b), refer to Chapter 13
7. d), refer to Chapters 13 and 14
8. c), refer to Chapter 6
9. a), refer to Chapter 9
10. b), refer to Chapter 9
11. b), refer to Chapter 14
12. c), refer to Chapter 13
13. c), refer to Chapters 2 and 3
14. a), refer to Chapter 13
15. d), refer to Chapter 6
16. d), refer to Chapter 6
17. a), refer to Chapter 6
18. a), refer to Chapter 6
19. c), refer to Chapter 19
20. a), refer to Chapter 19
21. c), refer to Chapter 21
22. a), refer to Chapter 21
23. b), refer Chapter 25
24. b), refer to Chapter 9
25. c), refer to Chapter 9
26. b), refer to Chapter 8
27. d), refer to Chapters 6 and 8
28. a), refer to Chapter 4
29. b), refer to Chapter 4
30. a), refer to Chapter 4
31. a), refer Chapter 4
32. a), refer Chapter 4
33. d), refer to Chapter 7
34. b), refer to Chapter 12
35. a), refer to Chapters 15 and 16
36. c), refer to Chapters 15 and 16
37. b), refer to Chapters 15 and 16
38. c), refer to Chapter 26
39. d), refer to Chapter 26
40. a), refer to Chapter 2
41. c), refer to Chapter 2
42. a), b), c), and d), refer Chapter 10
43. b), refer to Chapter 10
44. d), refer to Chapter 10
45. b), d), refer to Chapter 10
46. a), b), refer Chapter 18
47. a), refer Chapter 18
48. d), refer Chapter 22
49. b), refer Chapter 22
50. d), refer Chapter 23
51. c), refer to Chapter 5
52. a), refer Chapter 5
53. b, refer Chapter 24
54. a), refer Chapter 24
55. d), refer Chapters 5 and 24

Index

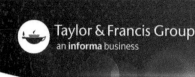

Milton Keynes UK
Ingram Content Group UK Ltd.
UKHW050827121223
434203UK00013B/144